Surekha Rathod
Vivek Harkare

Eustachian Tube Dysfunction and Its Impact on Hearing in OSMF

Surekha Rathod
Vivek Harkare

Eustachian Tube Dysfunction and Its Impact on Hearing in OSMF

Oral Submucous Fibrosis and Auditory Health: Exploring the Link with Eustachian Tube Dysfunction

LAP LAMBERT Academic Publishing

Imprint
Any brand names and product names mentioned in this book are subject to trademark, brand or patent protection and are trademarks or registered trademarks of their respective holders. The use of brand names, product names, common names, trade names, product descriptions etc. even without a particular marking in this work is in no way to be construed to mean that such names may be regarded as unrestricted in respect of trademark and brand protection legislation and could thus be used by anyone.

Cover image: www.ingimage.com

Publisher:
LAP LAMBERT Academic Publishing
is a trademark of
Dodo Books Indian Ocean Ltd. and OmniScriptum S.R.L publishing group

120 High Road, East Finchley, London, N2 9ED, United Kingdom
Str. Armeneasca 28/1, office 1, Chisinau MD-2012, Republic of Moldova, Europe
Managing Directors: Ieva Konstantinova, Victoria Ursu
info@omniscriptum.com

Printed at: see last page
ISBN: 978-620-8-43487-8

Contents

INTRODUCTION

Oral submucous fibrosis is a premalignant condition which occurs in Indians and South Asian countries[1].

The title atrophiaidiopathica (tropica) mucosa Oris 'was first described by Schwartz in 1952. Later idiopathic scleroderma of mouth, Sclerosing stomatitis and idiopathic palatal fibrosis used for this condition. This condition was first described separately in India, by Lal and Joshi in 1953 as diffuse oral submucous fibrosis 'and submucous fibrosis of the oral mucosa, palate and pillars etc.[1,2]

OSMF affects the oral mucosa, pharynx causing stiffness of the oral mucosa, vesicle formation and epithelial atrophy leading towards trismus.[3] The prevalence of OSMF in Indians is up to 0.4%, being highest in Southern India. It can be seen among all age groups of all socioeconomic strata and widely prevalent in India.[4] After the introduction of pan parag and gutkha etc into to the market, a sudden increase was noted in the incidence of OSMF.[5]

Etiopathogenesis:

The pathogenesis of OSMF has multifactorial etiology including nutritional deficiencies, ingestion of chillies, habit of chewing areca nut, factors like pollution and genetic and immunologic processes.

1. Chewing of Areca nut (betel nut):

The major component of betel quid is areca nut, tobacco, lime and piper leaf.

Betel nut is a major etiologic agent in OSMF.[6,7,8,9] Betel nut consists of arecoline, an active alkaloid which stimulates fibroblast to increase production of collagen by 150%[10] and also upregulates COX-2 expression[11]. It causes increased collagen production leading to fibrosis. Areca nut quid contains cytotoxic & genotoxic agents which leads to arecoline cytotoxicity and stimulates self-proliferation and thiol- depletion.[12]

Earlier studies have reported that, OSMF remains active even after termination of the chewing habit signifying that components of areca nut initiate OSMF. Gene expression in the fibroblasts is affected by areca nut, due to which greater amount of normal collagen is produced in OSMF[13].

Trivedy C et al. conducted a study and concluded that there is increased level of copper in saliva after placing a areca nut quid in mouth for 5- 10 min.[14] Copper stimulates fibrogenesis through up –regulation of lysyl oxidase activity by working as an initiating factor in OSMF.[15]

Table 1: Composition of some common names of arecanut[16]

Common names of Areca nut	Content of quid	Areas of consumption
Betel Quid	Areca nut alone or with lime. Areca nut dried alone or with lime.	South china, pacific island South Asia
Lao-hwa quid	Areca nut with lime and betel leaves.	Taiwan, China, Papua
Stem quid	Areca nut alone or with betel stem. Areca nut with leaves. Areca nut with lime and betel leaves.	Taiwan, china,
Paan or Pan	Areca nut with lime, tobacco , flavoring agent and betel leaves.	South Asia
Common form of Pan or Paan with tobacco	Areca nut with lime, flavoring agent and betel leaves.	South Asia, part of south-eastern Asia
Pan masala or chaalia	Areca nut with lime,other chemicals and flavoring agent.	India(paan masala), Pakistan (chaalia)
Mawa, Kharra	Areca nut with lime, other chemicals, tobacco, and flavoring agents.	India

2. Chilies.

One of the etiologies in OSMF is high content of chilly but it is controversial.

Sirsat (1960) reported that capsaicin is a major content of chilies which stimulated fibrosis of the palate in rats.[17]

3. Nutritional deficiencies:

Impaired healing of the inflamed oral mucosa occurs due to deficiencies like Iron deficiency anemia, vitamin B-complex deficiency, and malnutrition. This atrophic oral mucosa is more vulnerable to the chronic irritation from chilies and areca nut.

Ramnathan (1981) hypothesized that OSMF could be an Asian version of Sideropenic dysphagia based on his findings of prolonged vitamin B-complex and iron deficiency in Malaysian OSMFindividuals.[18]

4. Genetic and immunologic process:

Previous studies reported that pathogenesis of OSMF is genetic and immunologic process. The increased frequency of human leucocyte antigen DR3 (HLA-DR3) human leukocyte antigen A10. On the other hand, there are few individuals who showed genetic predisposition. Studies which are conducted recently reported that there are increased levels of proinflammatory cytokines and reduced antifibrotic interferon gamma (IFN-gamma) in OSMF individuals.[19]

5. Pollution:

Varghese et al (1986) conducted study on cashew workers of Kerala –south India and stated that there is a high incidence of OSMF in these population.[20]

The most common symptom of OSMF is burning sensation of the oral mucosa while taking hot and spicy food. Early symptoms of OSMF are vesiculation, ulceration, excessive salivation, recurrent stomatitis dryness of mouth and pigmentation. Characteristic of OSMF is fibrosis of buccal mucosa, mucosa of soft palate, lip mucosa and anterior pillars. They rarely involve the pharyngeal box, vocal cords, but is capable of involving the Eustachian tube. Various workers reported that OSMF affects the muscles of soft palate and subsequently may affect the Eustachian tube function.

Laboratory findings in individuals with OSMF include decreased hemoglobin, iron, vitamin B complex and protein levels; and increased erythrocyte sedimentation rate (ESR). Biopsy from affected oral site provides the definitive diagnosis.

Different treatment modalities are available for OSMF individuals, these treatments depend on the stages OSMF. In initial phase of the disease, stoppage of habit is the suitable choice of treatment. Even after treatment in severe cases it is irreversible. Role of steroids (topical or intralesional), placental extracts, hyaluronidase and interferon gamma (IFN-gamma) are still evolving. The severe cases of OSMF with trismus are managed by surgery and there is dysplastic changes seen histopathologically.

The definition of OSMF is chronic slowly progressive disease leading to fibrosis of oral mucosa causing restriction of jaw and tongue resulting in inability to eat and deglutition. OSMF is a multifactorial disease with an unknown etiology but the chronic irritation from fibers of areca nut may be the cause of OSMF.

Physiologically opening and closing of function of the Eustachian tube (ET) is important.[21] This ET is connected to middle ear cavity by nasopharynx. However, on normal opening of eustachian tube, the atmospheric pressure is equalized in middle ear whereas the closing of ET protects the middle ear from unwanted pressure fluctuations and loud sound. If there is impairment in closing and opening function of ET it leads to hearing disability due to changes in the middle ear.

In adults the ET is 36 mm long and is directed downwards, forwards and medially from the medial ear and consist of two parts; one portion i.e lateral third which is a bony portion of anterior wall of tympanic cavity,12 mm in size and a fibrocartilaginous portion which is 24mm in size i. e. medial 2/3rdentering the nasopharynx.

In OSMF the prominent features seen are involvement of soft palate muscle like tensor veli palatine and levator veli palatine. Numerous researchers have elaborated on the pathological changes of soft palate muscles.[21]

Hearing assessment.[22]

There are three types of hearing loss -

1. The conduction of sound from the external ear to the stapidio vestibular is called as conductive hearing loss. It is caused due to tympanic membrane perforate ion and ET tube obstruction and external ear obstruction.

2. In Sensorineural hearing loss, when the eight nerve lesions involved are termed as retrocochler and when the lesion with central auditory connection is known as central deafness.

3. Conductive and sensorineural deafness is termed as

mixed hearing loss. Mixed hearing loss present in some cases like chronic suppurative otitis media and otosclerosis.

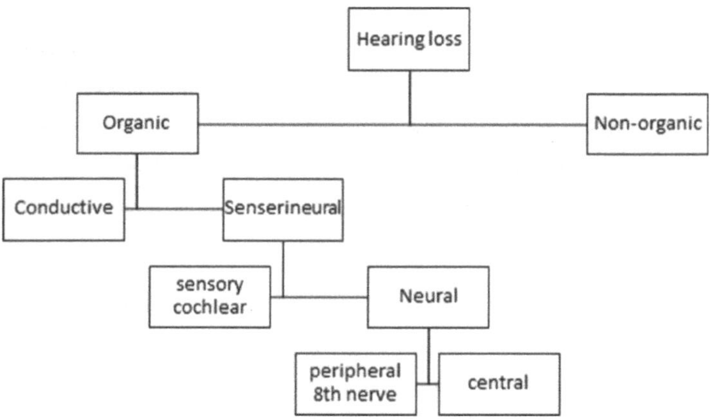

Figure 1: Types of Hearing Loss

The auditory function is assessed on[22]**-**

1. The sensorineural, conductive or mixed hearing loss

2. Mild hearing loss, moderate hearing loss, moderate to severe hearing loss, severe hearing loss and profound hearing loss.

3. Site of lesion- In conductive, the lesion might be present at tympanic membrane, external ear, middle ear, ossicle, eustachian tube, and ossicle in conductive hearing loss. We can find out these lesions by clinical elimination and tympanometry. If the lesions are cochlear, retrococlear or central then it is sensorineural.

4. Causes of hearing impairment can be traumatic, congenital, infective, degenerative, metabolic, is due to - the cause may be congenital, traumatic, infective, neoplastic, degenerative, metabolic, otitis, vascular/autoimmune process, so complete history taking and lab investigation is necessary.

Different methods for the assessment of hearing[22]

A. The Clinical test of assessment of hearing

1. Watch

2. Speech

3. finger

4. Tuning

i. Rinne test

ii. Weber test

iii. Absolute bone conduction test

iv. Schwabach's test

v. Bing test

vi. Gelle's test

B. Audiometric test-

Pure tone audiometric test (PTA) an audiometer is an electronic device the intensity of which can be increased or decreased in 5dB steps and it produces pure tones.

Usually air conduction threshold is measured fortunes of 125, 250, 500, 1000, 2000, 4000 and 8000 Hz and bone conduction threshold for 250, 500, 1000, 2000, 4000 Hz. The measure of the degree of hearing impairment is the amount of intensity that has to be raised above the normal level. The graph known as an audiogram is used for charting it. The measure of cochlear function is the threshold of bone conduction. The measure of the degree of conductive deafness is the difference in the threshold of air and bone conduction (A-B GAP)[22].

It may be noted that audiometer is so calibrated that the hearing of a normal person, both for air and bone conduction, is at 0 dB and there is no A-B GAP, while the tuning fork test normally show AC > BC.

The difference between the two ears is masked to avoid getting shadow curve from the non-test better ear. Similarly, masking is essential in all bone conduction studies. Masking is done by employing narrow band noise to non-test ear.

Uses of pure tone audiogram--

1. PTA is used to measure threshold of hearing by air and bone conduction.
2. PTA gives results in the form of graphs so for future references.
3. It is used for prescription of hearing aid.
4. Speech response threshold can be predicted.

OSMF has a multifactorial etiology and also there is a lack of response to current treatment modalities. In this condition research is needed to develop sensitive, specific and faster tests in the diagnosis and prognosis of these diseases. Trace elements like copper and zinc were found to have diagnostic and prognostic values in malignancies like lymphoma, carcinoma of lung, breast etc. Recently, trace elements are receiving a lot of attention in the detection of oral cancer and precancer as they were found to be significantly altered in these conditions.

TRACE ELEMENTS

The source of trace elements in humans can be through ingestion of food, water and soil or dermal absorption. The availability of trace elements in the humans depends upon the existence and non-existence of trace elements in the environment.[23]

History of metal toxicity and its treatment date back to 370 B.C.E with Hippocrates recording abdominal colic in a man working with extraction. Many other studies have reported metal toxicity of copper, mercury and lead in humans.[24]

In the second row sequence of periodic table and vanadium to zinc in the first row, the trace elements required for animal and plants include molybdenum. The concentration, absorption and persistence of the subsequent toxicant at the site of action of the metals determines its toxic effects. The reaction between final toxicants and endogenous target molecule severely alter the biological environment leads to toxic damage due the structural and functional changes.[24]

Heightening of the Oxidative processes result in the increase of hydrogen peroxide and superoxide anion radical that form a base for other connections with signaling response.[24]

Investigations into the function of elements present in minute amount in tissue has been hampered by insensitive quantitative methods.[25] With the advent of such techniques as Atomic Absorption Spectrophotometry (AAS), it becomes possible to study the role of certain trace elements. Today zinc, copper, iron, cobalt, selenium and molybdenum comprise the list of trace elements identified in all types of living organisms. Present evidence suggests that deficiency of one of these is associated with the syndrome of series of pathological changes reflecting structural and thus, presumably underlying physiological, biological and metabolic disturbances. Subsequent administration of missing elements results in partial or complete remission of deficiency signs, depending upon the degree and the nature of cellular damage associated with the deficiency state. Copper, zinc and iron are the trace elements whose major biological effects in various pathological conditions have been recently studied.

COPPER

Physiology of Copper Historical background:

Copper (Cu), one of the most used metallic elements discovered about 8000.

B.C. has been of interest to physicians for many hundred years and of late it plays an important role in investigative evaluation[26].Copper was recognized as a regular constitute of human blood in 1875.[27]

Body copper distribution

100 to 150 mg of copper is contained in adult body. The distribution of Cu in the body is as follows;

Muscles - 64 mg

Bone - 23mg

Liver - 18mg

Blood - 90mg/dl in serum (on an average)

Liver contains a higher concentration of copper than any other organ studied. The concentration of Cu in the fetal liver is five to ten times higher than that in the liver of an adult. Hence, this may serve as a compensation for the period during which the sole diet of the infant is milk which is relatively low in copper. The levels of copper in the liver of an infant requires around five to fifteen years to crop to the adult level. A large part of the total body copper i.e about 50% to 70% is found in the muscles and bones.

Both the blood cells and serum contain copper. In red blood cells Cu content remain constant while that of the serum is variable in the range of 70 mg/dl to 140 mg/dl. 60% of copper in red blood cells occur as erythrocuprein and the remaining 40% as non-erythrocuprein form.[28] Copper in plasma occurs in two main forms, one firmly bound and the other loosely bound. The firmly bound copper comprising about 80% to 90% of the total plasma copper is made up of ceruloplasmin. Ceruloplasmin, a copper binding plasma protein, has molecular weight of about 18000 and contains 0.34% Cu about 8 atoms of copper/mole.30 mg of Ceruloplasmin is present per deciliter of normal plasma. The loosely bound copper is called ―direct reacting‖ copper because it reacts freely with copper complexing reagents (eg. Dithizon and diethyldithiocarbamate) and is loosely bound to protein, probably serum albumin. The albumin bound copper may represent the copper in transport.[29] 9.5 mg/g to 11.3 mg/g of Copper has been found in human teeth.[30]

Requirements and sources:

The human requirement of copper has been studied by balance experiments.

The daily allowance of copper is suggested as follows:

Adults- 2.5 mg.[29]

Infants & children - 0.05 mg/kg body weight.[28]

This is easily supplied in an average diet which contains 2.5 mg to 5.0 mg of copper. Copper is widely distributed in the food items; most diets provide the amount needed per day to maintain copper balance.

The richest sources of dietary copper are:

Liver 44.1 mg

Nuts 11.6 mg

Legumes 9.0 mg

Cereals 4.7 mg

Fruits 9.2 mg

Poultry 3.0 mg

Fish 2.5 mg

Green legumes 1.7 mg

Leafy vegetables 1.2 mg

Cow's milk is a poor source of copper (concentration of 0.015 mg/dl to 0.18 mg/dl). Human milk contains copper ranging from 1.015 mg/dl at the beginning of lactation to 0.15 mg/dl at the end.[28]

Absorption and metabolism

Absorption of copper mainly occurs from stomach and proximal intestine. Dietary copper is poorly absorbed. From intestine, copper passes to plasma and is distributed to liver, red blood corpuscles and other tissues. Copper excretion occurs mainly through urine, milk, sweat and menstrual flow.[31]

The small but characteristic amount of copper present in the blood is distributed equally between Red blood corpuscles and plasma.[27] The copper-carrying glycoprotein, Ceruloplasmin curbs the occurrence of toxic iron products by ferric oxidase activity. Also, it controls the oxidation of membrane lipid.[32] A good association is seen between ceruloplasmin levels and the oxidative activity.[27] The remainder of plasma copper is found loosely bound to albumin (direct reacting fraction). Cellular copper is primarily found in mitochondria.33 Remainder of body copper is mainly incorporated into various kinds of copper storage proteins such as erythrocytes in the RBC and the cerebrocuprum in the liver.[29]

Experiments have been carried out with labeled copper. Copper was found to be largely associated with the albumin fraction of the plasma immediately after its ingestion. A decline in plasma radioactivity occurs, as copper attached to albumin is distributed to cuproprotein in the liver and elsewhere, a secondary rise in plasma radioactivity then takes place as copper present in ceruloplasmin of liver is released in the blood. Since copper in the plasma is largely bound to protein, it is not readily excreted in the urine. Most of it is excreted via bile into the intestine and expelled with faeces.[28]

Functions

1. In several proteins, metalo-enzymes and some naturally occurring pigments copper is present as a necessary constituent.[31]

2. Several evidences points out to a role in the hemoglobin synthesis or hematopoiesis as the main function of copper, the exact nature of which is unknown (Sachs et al, 1935). Hemocyanin is a copper protein complex in the blood of certain invertebrates, where it functions like hemoglobin, as an oxygen carrier enzyme.[28]

3. There are two key enzymes that contain copper as a chief constituent; cytochrome C-oxidase, responsible for the major part (more than 90% probably) of the oxygen consumed by life on this planet and superoxide dismutase of the cytosol. This enzyme acts as a catalyst for scavenging of the toxic free radical superoxide ion O produced during aerobic metabolism. Cytosolic superoxide dismutase has a molecular weight of 32,000 and it consists of two identical subunits and contains one Cu and one zinc subunit (Fredovich, 1975).[28]

4. Copper is essential for maintenance of myelin sheath of the nervous system and normal bone formation.[29]

5. It is related with the activity of tyrosinase enzyme, catalase, delta amino levulimic acid hydrase in porphyrins synthesis.[29]

6. Vascular and structural integrity: Copper is concerned with cross-linkage bounding (amino oxidase) of collagen and elastin, thus giving stability to arteries and bones.[31]

7. By playing an important role in myelogenesis and catecholamine metabolism, copper helps in maintaining of the structure as well as function of central nervous system.[28]

Deficiency

Factors predisposing to copper deficiency in the body:

1. Dietary factors: deficiency of copper may be due to low intake of copper in the diet as is usually seen in infants or due to malabsorption.

2. Genetically acquired defect in copper absorption or the primary defect or the synthesis of an abnormal protein (copper thiamine) which is inherited as an autosomal recessive pattern can be the cause of defect in copper metabolism in the body.[31]

Hypocupremia:

1. Hypocupremia have been reported in malabsorption (kwashiorkor, celiac diseases, sprue), miasmic infants and nephritic syndrome.[31]

2. Two clinical syndromes due to dietary copper deficiency have been reported in infants.

i. One of the syndromes is characterized by moderate to severe anemia, low serum iron and copper levels, which are responsive to the combined copper and iron therapy. This syndrome is seen in infants fed with low copper milk diet.

ii. Bone changes and hypocupremia seen in syndromes like anemia, recurrent diarrhea and scurvy. This syndrome is seen in infants rehabilitated on high caloric and low copper diet.

3. Two disorders of metabolic errors associated with copper metabolism have been reported. They are:

i. Menke's kinky hair syndrome is characterized by genetic defect in copper absorption, seen in infants, subnormal copper level in blood, liver and hair, metaphyseal lesions and degenerative changes in aortic elastin.

ii. Wilson's disease (Hepatolenticular degeneration) is characterized by in co-ordination of ataxia, progressive mental deterioration, post necrotic cirrhosis with excessive copper deposition in the liver, brain, cornea, kidneys, together with low serum ceruloplasmin level, high urinary copper level and reduced faecal excretion of copper. The primary defect is in the synthesis of abnormal protein (copper thiamine) with a high affinity of copper.

Hypercupremia:

1. Elevated serum copper is reported to be physiological in pregnancy[29] and following administration of estrogens[33](whether as oral contraceptives or for other reasons) or thyroid and pituitary hormones and after surgery.[27]

2. Acute poisoning by copper is characterized by metallic taste, salivation[31] burning pain in the stomach, vomiting, diarrhea, hematuria, uremia and jaundice[34] (in severe cases). In large dosages circulatory collapse occurs. Paralysis of limbs, coma and death may also occur.[31]

3. Chronic poisoning is due to prolonged exposure to fumes of copper in industries, consumption of food kept in copper utensils.[3] It is characterized by the purple line on the gums, diarrhea, bronchitis, renal damage, anemia, peripheral neuritis and atrophy of muscles. Direct contact with skin can cause dermatitis and eczematous lesions.[34]

4. An increased copper level in the serum has been reported in various pathological conditions such as multiple sclerosis, myocardial infarctions, acute and chronic liver diseases, schizophrenia, congestive cardiac failure, thyrotoxicosis, rheumatic heart disease, anemia and various malignancies.

5. In Indian childhood cirrhosis hepatic, serum and urinary copper is much higher than normal individuals. The exact cause of raised hepatic concentration is not known.

Hypercupremia may be due to[31]:-

Excessive ingestion and absorption of copper in the form of Ayurvedic and traditional medicines given to infants and pregnant mothers.

i) Liver cell necrosis with release of copper in circulation.

ii) Anemia due to non-utilization of copper.

iii) Acute and chronic infections.

iv) Raised estrogen levels.

v) Increase in ceruloplasmin. It is not clear whether raised hepatic and serum copper is an ex an expression of primary, inherited metabolic defect peculiar to Indian children or it represents a secondary event. Therapy of Indian childhood cirrhosis individuals with chelating agents such as penicillamine is still in conclusive.

Biological mechanism in carcinogenesis:

The mechanism underlying the elevation of copper level in malignancies is not clear. Underwood (1956) postulates that in Hodgkin's disease and probably on other malignant states, the intestinal barrier to copper level is lowered, leading to a rapid absorption by the liver where more ceruloplasmin is formed and released into the circulation. This supports the suggestion by Shields et.al (1969) and Shifrine et.al (1976) that hypercupremia is the result of an increase in the concentration of circulating ceruloplasmin, which is the copper protein in vertebrate plasma.[35,36]

It was also suggested that the elevation of copper level in malignancy is due to the destruction and necrosis of tissues leading to the release of copper present in the affected tissue into the circulation.[29] The liver is the largest store house of copper in the body, other organs rich in copper been the bones and the brain, the common sites for metastases. This could be the possible factor for much higher serum copper level in individuals with hepatic metastasis and in those with widely disseminated cancers with secondaries in bones or brain in turn causing extensive necrosis of the tissues and thus releasing large amount of copper into blood.[37]

Free radicals particularly superoxide radicals, have been incriminated as a possible cause of cancer. Trace levels of copper dramatically enhance the biological damage caused by superoxide radicals. The involvement of copper ions in biological damage caused by superoxide, a radical found in all living tissues has recently been documented. According to this model, superoxide reduced the copper in the cells to the cuprous state. The cuprous ions react with hydrogen peroxide to form hydroxyl radical that damage proteins, ribonucleic acid and most importantly deoxy-ribonucleic acid. Repetitive formation of hydroxyl radicals where the copper ions are found, is probably the mechanism of this process in the nuclei. The radicals may cause double strands breaks in the nuclear DNA that are not repairable, thus initiating a malignant process. Since most of the copper found in the tissues is specifically bound comprising an integral part of various enzymes, a slight increase in total tissue copper concentration may represent a considerable increase in the non-specific complexed copper, that by itself is responsible for biological damage.[38]

ZINC

Physiology of Zinc:

Historical Background:

The biological role of zinc was first established over hundred years back by Raultin 1869, but it was not until 1939, that zinc deficiency was indicated in vitamin deficiency states such as beri-beri. Research during the past two decades has shown the importance of zinc in biologic and metabolic activities of man. Extensively documented zinc is recognized to be fundamental to life.[29]

Body-Zinc Distribution:

Zinc (Zn) is widely distributed in the tissues of the body. The body zinc pool is1.40 mg to 2.39 mg. The zinc distribution in the body is as follows:

Skin	:	90µg/g to 250 µg/g
Bone	:	90µg/g to 250 µg/g
Blood	:	10 µg/g to 14 µg/g (erythrocytes)
Liver	:	140 µg/g to 230 µg/g
Kidney	:	140 µg/g to 230 µg/g
Nails	:	90µg/g to 250 µg/g

Requirement and Sources:

Table 2: Daily requirement of zinc:

Infants :	0 to 3 months	0.70 mg to 3 mg
Children :	6 to 12 months	3 mg to 5mg
Children: Preadolescents		6 mg to 10mg
Adolescents:		8 mg to 13 mg
Adults: Men and women		10 mg to 20 mg
Pregnant women		25 mg to 35 mg
Lactating mother		20 mg to 25 mg

Metabolic studies have shown that in healthy adults an intake of 8.00 mg to 10.00 mg per day is sufficient to bring about equilibrium with respect to zinc. The currently recommended allowance is 15.00 mg/day. The daily requirement of zinc is dependent on many factors: both physiological and environmental. Pregnancy, lactation and periods of growth are just some of these factors.

A problem of low zinc concentration has been described in North American children in Denver, Colorado, with an associated loss of taste and smell acuity. Hamgbridge et al found that substantial sections of the US population may suffer from marginal zinc deficiency. Zinc deficiency is reported in countries like Egypt and Iran, where malabsorption occurs because of phytate ingestion. This is probably responsible for a syndrome comprising anemia, hepatosplenomegaly and hypogonal dwarfism.

Diet is the principal source of zinc. A balanced diet containing sufficient animal protein should provide the daily zinc allowance. Meat, liver, eggs, seafood (particularly crysters), milk and whole grains products are good sources. Unlike other trace elements like iron, there are substantial body-store reserves of zinc for mobilization. This highlights the need for an adequate intake of zinc.[29]

The microminerals are constant ingredients of human teeth.39 Zinc has been reported from a level of between 194 g/ml of human whole teeth and up to 200 g/ml in enamel surface.[40] The mean level of Zn of dentin in human teeth has been reported to be 174.7 ppm by Derise and Ritchey.39 Above 75% of the zinc found in saliva is contained in parotid protein gustin'.

Absorption and metabolism

In normal conditions most of the dietary zinc is excreted in the faeces and only a small portion of it is absorbed.[41] Zinc is absorbed throughout the intestine. The most rapid accumulation and turnover rate of zinc occurs in soft tissues especially the pancreas, liver, kidneys and spleen. Liver crystal contains zinc-copper binding proteins which may serve as storage protein for zinc. Amount of zinc deposits present in bones are comparatively large, however with the rest of the organism these stores do not move into rapid circulation equilibrium. The body pool of biologically available zinc appears to be small and have a rapid turnover.[29] However, long period of varying dietary zinc supplies lead to adaptive changes in intestinal absorption and the body compensates for it by adjusting to endogenous secretion. Only very small amounts are excreted in the urine and sweat; however, the latter may appreciably be higher in hot climate.[41]

Function

Zinc is an important element is for the normal growth, reproduction and life expectancy of animals and human beings and has a beneficial effect on the process of repair of tissue & wound healing.[42]

a. Zinc and enzymes: Prasad stated that zinc is required by over 70 metallo- enzymes for their proper function. Most recently Kay asserted that the number of metallo-enzymes dependent on zinc are closer to 100. For alcoholic metabolism, alcohol dehydrogenase needed. The cell proliferation, replication and differentiation are essential for DNA and RNA polymerase and carboxypeptidase for protein digestion.[42]

b. Zinc and tissue metabolism: It is believed that zinc stimulates fibroblasts via DNA synthesis to produce collagen and promote scar formation. Consequently, zinc has been used as a post-operative supplement and as a topical agent in suitably impregnated surgical tapes.42 Zinc is necessary to maintain concentration of vitamin A in plasma. It may be required for metabolism of vitamin A from the liver. When vitamin A concentration in the plasma is lower than normal and patient is unresponsive to therapy with vitamin A, zinc supplementation may be effective.[28]

In studies on rats, Chausmer et al, demonstrated an apparent tissue specific influence exerted on zinc homeostasis by the hormone calcitonin. Calcitonin synthesis by the _C _cells of the thyroid gland is activated by zinc. In very sophisticated studies, using neutron activation analyses, Japanese investigators have demonstrated the presence of zinc in all tissues, with the highest concentration seen in the liver, the assembly site for metallo-enzymes.[42]

c. Zinc and taste: About 75% of the zinc in saliva is contained in the parotid protein gustin. Shutzman and associates speculated that gustin and/or zinc is important to maintain normal taste activity. They conceived that the other factors including hormones, other trace elements, neurotransmitters also play a role in taste and olfaction. Furthermore, they state that even individuals with normal levels of salivary zinc often exhibit severe hypogeusia. Nevertheless, it is documented that oral administration of zinc sulphate can lead to partial recovery of taste acuity.[42,43]

Driezen and associates state that individuals given prophylactic zinc prior to radiation therapy to salivary glands have fewer gustatory complaints and less severe hypogeusia. Damage to the microvilli and outer surface of the taste buds have been proposed as the principal site of taste loss following radiation therapy.[42]

d. Zinc and immune system: Dietary zinc supplementation has been shown by researchers to improve T-cell abnormalities. Conversely, in experiment with mice, Fernandes and co-workers have shown that dietary zinc produced immunologic abnormalities of both T and B cells. Tumor immunity, a T cell function may be impaired by low serum zinc level.[42]

Cunninghan-Ruddles et al have demonstrated that zinc is a B-cell mitogen, a substance which stimulates mitosis. The tumor immunity improves by reducing production of B cell blocking factors. These findings also seen to support the conclusions of Mathur and Wallenius.[42]

e. Zinc or zinc compounds as drugs: Zinc sulfate has shown some promise in the treatment of Herpes simplex infections. Zinc ions, in vitro, have been shown to inhibit virus replication.[42]

Hypozincaemia

Factors predisposing to zinc deficiency:

i. Dietary factors: Although the diet may contain a sufficient amount of zinc, some food items contain dietary factors which affect the absorption of zinc, Phytate, a phosphate rich component found predominantly in cereals and fibers is one of these factors. It binds with zinc, forming complexes which reduce bioavailability of zinc. Other dietary factors affecting zinc absorption are calcium, milk and cheese.

ii. Inter-element competition: Inter-element competition with simultaneous oral administration of iron as a dietary supplement can also affect zinc bioavailability.

iii. Hypozincemia or low serum zinc levels is a nonspecific observation. Among the causes of zinc deficiency Prasad lists alcohol consumption, liver diseases, gastro intestinal disorders, renal diseases, neoplasia, burns and dermatoses, parasitic infections, collagen disorders, pregnancy disorders, genetic disorders, diseases producing increasing muscle metabolism and acute tissue injury. Steroid therapy administration of post-operative contraceptives also producehypozincaemia.[29]

Clinical manifestation of zinc deficiency -

The clinical signs of acute zinc deficiency as described by Kay include apathy, confusion, mental depression as well as inflammatory changes which begin in oral mucosa and nasolabial fold areas. These changes progress rapidly to involve the orifices and extremities.[42] Clayton B.C. in her review of trace elements found that changes due to zinc deficiency are impaired brain growth, anorexia, growth retardation, hypogonadism and delayed sexual maturity, alopecia, skin changes such as acrodermatitis enteropathy, skeletal changes, diarrhea and infection susceptibility. Both Prasad and Clayton agree that malabsorption problems play a vital role in zinc deficiency.

Hyperzincaemia:

The workers who work in galvanizer and molten brass industry causes. The acute symptoms are similar to an anaphylactic response. These responses include nausea, vomiting, fever, sweating, pulse rate high, burning and dryness of upper respiratory tract. Chronic zinc stomatitis is characterized by congestion and suppuration of the gingival tissues with bluish grey line and metallic taste. The teeth may becomeloose due to destruction of alveolar process, although little pain is experienced. However, salivary glands are involvement seen and submaxillary lymph node was painful.[43]

Biological mechanism in carcinogenesis:

In human cancer role of Zn is not known Chuapil has proposed that zinc is the integral part of trio membrane. It may be involved in the stability of membranes, also control membrane integrity. Zinc has been observed to function as nitrogen including blastogen transformation of lymphocytes in a fashion similar to that of phytohemagglutinin. Phytohemagglutinin effects are also greater in lymphocytes harvested from rats that had been given a high zinc diet.

In RNA and DNA polymerase zinc causes inhibitory effect on cell membrane bound adenyl cyclase in carcinogenesis. Zinc has also been shown to stabilize ribosomes and the DNA double helix, Bharadwaj and Luthra[36] who conducted a study on hamster cheek pouch for oral carcinogenesis. He observed that during progressive carcinogenesis, DNA activity was high hence zinc is essential for DNA synthesis Mutch Haualey stated that zinc impaired cell differentiation and DNA synthesis.

Mcquity et al[30] suggested the following possible explanation for the observed decreased levels of zinc in sera or cells from human cancer individuals. The serum zinc may be low because the element is selectively used by the tumor at the expense of the host. Zinc levels may be low in cancer cells compared with normal because the available zinc is divided among the cells competing for it. Dennes et al have observed an inverse correlation between leukemia cell content and leucocyte zinc content.[44] Whether zinc depletion could occur in this way is not clear. Davies et al state that no correlation could be made between decreased plasma zinc and the growth and spread of neoplasm.[45]

Fernandes and co-workers have shown that dietary zinc restriction produced immunologic abnormalities of both T and B- cells.[46]

Tumor immunity, a T-cell function may be impaired by low serum zinc levels. A lower concentration of zinc in crystal, in combination with suitable concentration of copper, might inhibit protein synthesis. There is a considerable lowering of the enzymatic capacities to remove free O2 radicals; it is possible that paradoxid dismutase synthesis may be impaired by zinc deficiency in the malignant cells. Cunnigham-Ruddlesetal have demonstrated that zinc is a B-cell mitogen. A substance which stimulates mitosis. In recent research demonstrated that for proper regulation of genome activity and cell cycle by acidic nuclear protein. Nucleo histones are the major fractions of nuclear proteins. The nucleo histones are reduced in zinc deficiency.[33]

Mathur et al reported that diet which content added zinc delays the zinc influences carcinogenesis in two ways. Supplementary zinc postpones delays the onset of carcinogenesis. However, diet which is low content of zinc causes initial changes histologically.[46]

IRON

Iron deficiency is most prevalent deficiency in India. Total iron content of normal adult is about 4 to 5gms. It is present and distributed in the body in various forms as[33]

	Compound/forms	Function
A)	Haem Iron	
1.	Hemoglobin, Myoglobin	O2 carrier
2.	Cytochromes	Electron carrier
3.	Peroxidase	Peroxide breakdown
4.	Catalase	
B)	Non-Haem Iron	
1.	Transferrin	

Transport of iron

2.	Lactoferrin	
3.	Ferritin and haemosiderin	Storage of iron
4.	Flavoproteins, dehydrogenase	Oxidizing enzymes and oxidases

The recommended daily allowance of iron for an adult Indian is 20mg. Children between 13-15 years need 20-30mg/day, whereas pregnant women need 40mg/day.[47,48]

The richest dietary source of iron is animal viscera e.g. liver, kidney, heart and spleen. Other good sources egg yolks, fish, oysters, dates, dried legumes. As the body conserves iron extremely well, only 6 to 12% of dietary intake needs to be absorbed in order to maintain iron equilibrium. However, iron deficiency states develop during growth, pregnancy or pathological conditions.[49,50,51]

Iron is absorbed from the upper part of duodenum. Ferric ions present in food are reduced with the help of gastric HCl, ascorbic acid, cysteine and –SH groups of proteins.

Iron absorption is decreased by phytate (present in cereals), oxalate (in leafy vegetables) and phosphates by forming insoluble iron salts. Tea and eggs also inhibit absorption to a lesser extent. Alcohol ingestion favors, whereas copper deficiency decreases iron absorption.[52]

Iron metabolism is unique as homeostasis is maintained by regulation at the level of absorption and not by excretion. Only small fraction of iron in the intestinal lumen enters the mucosal cell in the ferrous state. This binds with an intracellular carrier protein initially and then transfer the iron to apoferritin. The ferritin thus formed is kept temporarily in the mucosal cell. If there is anemia, the iron is transported into blood stream in combination with transferrin; otherwise the iron remaining in the mucosal cell is lost when the cell is desquamated. In blood, ceruloplasmin (ferroxidase 1) oxidizes ferrous to ferric state.

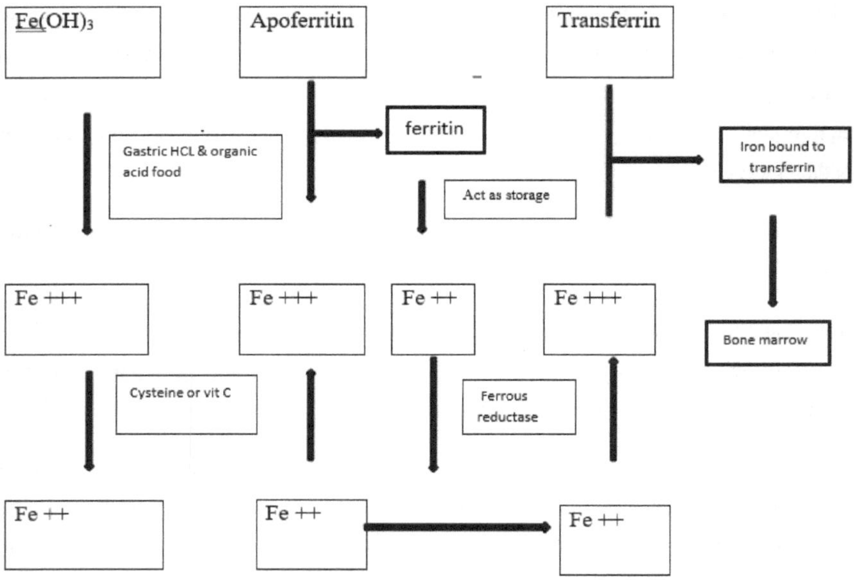

Figure 2: Diagrammatic representation of iron absorption and transport metabolism[5]

Iron level in serum shows diurnal variation; maximum level is attained in the morning and decreases slowly throughout the day. The average serum iron level is about 125 µg/dl in females. There is no seasonal variation in iron levels. In the elderly, the serum iron level decreases to 40 to 80 µg/dl.

Serum iron is elevated in pathologic states like:

1) Conditions of increased erythrocyte destruction (hemolytic anemia).

2) Decreased blood formation (lead poisoning or pyridoxine deficiency).

3) Increased release of iron from the body store (release of ferritin in acute hepatic cell necrosis).

4) Defective iron storage (pernicious anemia), and

5) Increased rate of absorption (hemochromatosis and transfusion siderosis, nutritional siderosis).

Decreased serum iron occurs in association with:

- Generalised iron deficiency (lack of sufficient dietary iron, inadequate absorption or chronic loss as a result of bleeding or nephrosis)
- Impaired release of iron from reticuloendothelial system (in infection), malignancy, and rheumatoid arthritis.

Iron deficiency results in decreased work capacity and productivity, behavioral changes, impaired lymphocyte transformation, reduce bacterial activity of neutrophils and impaired DNA synthesis.[47]

Only minute amounts of iron are excreted in the urine, faeces and sweat. Iron is also lost from the skin by means of sweating, hair loss and nail clippings.[54]

Rationale

The search for potential markers associated with severity as well as the susceptibility of OSMF, has been receiving considerable attention. Although role of many other trace element evaluated in OSMF but effect of OSMF on Eustachian tube dysfunction in OSMF is still undermined. The basic rational of the research was to evaluate and compare the effect of OSMF on Eustachian tube dysfunction and correlate the Cu, Zn and Fe with Eustachian tube dysfunction in OSMF and to predict future degree of Eustachian tube dysfunction.

The OSMF is slowly progressive pre-cancerous condition affecting oral mucosa and mostly found in younger generation. In India and south east Asian countries have high prevalence of OSMF. It is chronic disease affecting oral mucous membrane, fibro elastic changes of juxta epithelial layer inflammatory reaction and characterized by rigidity in mucosa causing partial trismus. However, previous studies reported OSMF affects parts of oral cavity including oral mucosa, soft palate, hard palate, pharynx and Eustachian tube. Physiologically opening and closing of function of ET is important. This ET is connected to middle ear cavity by nasopharynx. However, on normal opening of ET, the atmospheric pressure is equalized in middle ear whereas the closing of ET protects the middle ear from unwanted pressure fluctuations and loud. If there is impairment in closing and opening function of ET it leads to hearing disability due to changes in the middle ear.

The muscles attached to ET are tensor veli palatine and levator veli palatine muscles called as paratubal muscles. ET is a dynamic organ and cartilaginous in nature. ET function is impaired when surrounding muscle structures are involved.

The method which are commonly used to differentiate healthy mucosa from OSMF affected mucosa are clinical and histopathologic method. However, these methods have inherent limitation that the disease condition is diagnosed with a delayed stage and progression of once the patient develops OSMF then it requires extensive treatment including non-surgical and surgical therapy, which in some cases turns into malignancy and requires extensive chemotherapy and surgical therapy. All this increases treatment time as well as cost of treatment, this increases overall burden on the treatment. Hence, it is advantageous to forecast the future disease activity at an earlier stage, by knowing the exact stage of OSMF and Eustachian tube dysfunction and levels of Cu, Zn, Fe of OSMF. This level helps in providing appropriate and minimum treatment at an initial stage of OSMF and hearing impairment and reversal of disease condition by proper interceptive measures.

However, most of the currently used methods do not accurately predict the conversion of healthy mucosa to OSMF at initial level from OSMF to cancer.

A biomarker-based method would be appropriate to evaluate positive point at which levels of trace elements and OSMF and hearing loss. Many biomarkers have been evaluated in the previous studies in healthy, OSMF and cancer.

Trace elements are one of the biomarkers. Due to their vast pro and anti- inflammatory and antioxidant effects, trace elements have been implicated in various disease processes. However, the amount of trace element is important for function of the body and needs minimum quantity.Various trace elements have been studied for their possible uses as the diagnostic and prognostic tool for OSMF.

The limited amount of work in relation to trace elements and Eustachian tube dysfunction in OSMF patient. Warrants Future investigation to confirm diagnostic and prognostic guidelines for association of Eustachian dysfunction leading to hearing impairment and levels of trace elements in OSMF patient. All the studies evaluating the levels of biomarkers in serum have found that the Cu levels to be increased and Fe and Zn levels to be decreased in OSMF individuals. However, none of the studies have evaluated the Eustachian tube dysfunction leading to hearing loss and level of Cu, Zn, Fe in individuals with and without OSMF group.

Therefore, the current literature search was conducted evaluate and compare the Eustachian tube dysfunction leading to hearing impairment and levels of trace elements in with and without OSMF group. So as to find out its possible use as diagnostic and prognostic marker.

Teenagers and youths are getting more attracted to commercially available betel nut which are available in market in the form of Gutkha, pan masala, etc. There was strong association between areca nut and OSMF. Areca nut causes fibroblast stimulation, proliferation and collagen synthesis.

Various studies have been done on OSMF pathological changes, in the muscles of the soft palate. Degenerative changes, edematous muscle fibers and atrophy in palatal and para tubal muscles have been reported. Involvement of these muscles subsequently may affect the function of Eustachian tube.

There is a scarcity of information related to the involvement of the Eustachian tube and Para tubal muscles due to OSMF irrespective of numerous studies of OSMF reporting fibrosis and hyalinization in the sub-epithelium. Involvement of these muscles subsequently may affect the function of Eustachian tube.

There are number of studies conducted on oral submucous fibrosis and its effect on surrounding tissues but little information related to the association of the Eustachian tube dysfunction in OSMF.

REVIEW OF LITERATURE

Systematic review strategy

The rate of oral submucous fibrosis in India is 1% transformation risk. OSMF is a premalignant condition which affects any part of oral and characterized by vesicle formation, burning sensation, inability to eat causes epithelial atrophy leading to difficulty in opening the jaw cavity.[2]

Historically, OSMF was prevalent in even in days of shusrutha and termed as Vidari. Atrophia Idiopathica mucosa gave termed by Schwartz in 1952 which was found in five east African women of Indian origin. However, termed oral submucous fibrosis by Joshi in 1953.[55]

The etiology of this disease is multifactorial which includes genetic, betel nut chewing, ingestion of chilies, immunologic process, nutritional deficiency and pollution.[56] The major arecanut alkaloid are areoline, arecadine, arecolidine, guyacoline and guacine.[57]

Figure 3: Prisma Flow Chart

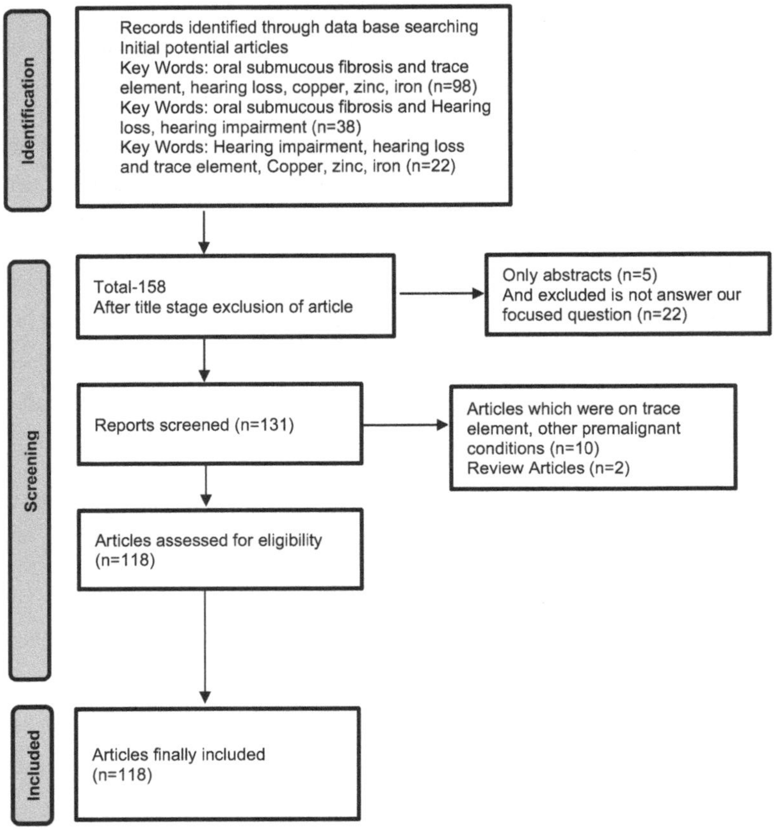

Trace elements are compounds that are essential in small amount for maintaining the integrity of physiological and metabolic mechanism within the body. It is required as essential component of biological enzyme system or biologically active constituents in structural portions. The essential trace elements like Cu, Iron and Zinc are necessary for immune function, normal growth and development.

Modulating effect of trace elements in predisposition of oral malignant condition have been recently documented. Elevated serum copper levels in OSMF has an initiating role as it stimulates fibrogenesis by upregulation of lysyl oxidase, thereby causing inhibition of degradation of collagen.[58]

Decrease level of zinc in OSMF causes upregulation COX-2 which enhances proliferation of cell, inhibits apoptosis and modulates angiogenesis which eventually leads to carcinogenesis and decrease in iron content result from uptake of iron in collagen synthesis and decreases epithelial vascularity leading to elevation of penetration of arecoline and which ultimately leads to fibrosis.[58]

By definition hearing is transduction of sound to neural impulses and its interpretation by the CNS and hearing loss means defect at any level from sound transduction to interpretation i.e. the ability to hear is reduced. There is a fibrosis of palatal causes ET dysfunction leading to conductive hearing loss in OSMF. Also, some author confirmed the study and reported that, involvement of pharyngeal orifice and nasopharynx.[59]

Considering the paramount literature available and for the ease of understanding, the review of literature has been segregated into two parts:

1. **Oral submucous fibrosis and hearing status.**
2. **Oral submucous fibrosis and trace elements.**

ORAL SUBMUCOUS FIBROSIS AND HEARING STATUS

SC Gupta in(2004)[60], carried out a study on 53 cases of OSMF (106 ears) for the assessment of ET function with tympanometry. Normal type-A curve showed in 80 ears. Abnormal tympanograms included type-B curves in 17(16%) and type-C curve in 9 (85%) ears. On testing the compliance of middle ear there was a shift in the compliance peaks in 78 (73.6%) ears with +200 daPa pressure change indicating normal Eustachian tube functions. In 28 (26.4%) ears, Eustachian tube functions were found to be affected as there was no shift in compliance peaks similarly on -200 daPa pressure change in 24 (22.7%) ears there was no shift in compliance peak. Hence, it was concluded that OSMF affects the ET function.

Shah et al (2011)[61], conducted a study to evaluate the effect of OSMF on ET function on 27 OSMF individuals and 25 normal individuals. All the individuals were screened by ET function test. Out of the 54 ears in the OSMF group 77.7% ears showed type A curve,22.2% ears have type-C curve and type -B curve was absent whereas in normal individuals 92% ears showed type-A curve, 4% ear have type- B curve and type-C curve found in 4% ears. The study concluded that OSMF causes the ET dysfunction.

Chaudhary MS et al (2013)[21] conducted a cross sectional study to determine hearing loss in OSMF individuals. It comprised of 20 individuals with OSMF, a detailed case history taken and all individuals were screened for pure tone audiometry. In grade I OSMF individuals hearing loss in right and left sides. Individuals with grade II OSMF bilateral hearing loss in five patients whereas in grade III individuals had bilateral mild conductive hearing loss. Grade III OSMF patients had bilateral mild CHL. There was a significant correlation seen with OSMF and hearing loss.

Siddiqui SN et al (2014)[62], evaluated ET function and its correlation with grades of OSMF. It consisted of 20 OSMF individuals (40 ears) and 20 normal individuals (40 ears). All OSMF and normal individuals underwent audiometry test and tympanometry analysis showed no statistically significant differences seen when compared in OSMF and normal individuals. However, in OSMF individuals showed a statistically significant difference in eustachian tube function in OSMF individuals. The present study concluded that the amount of deviation found in ET function, it does not contribute to cause of hearing deficit.

Devi P et al (2015)[63], evaluated the hearing loss in OSMF individuals. A study consisted of 40 individuals with OSMF and 10 normal individuals. Both groups were evaluated by pure tone audiometry. The OSMF group showed a significant degree of hearing loss as compared with normal individuals and concluded that mild conductive hearing loss existed in OSMF individuals

Badra S et al (2015)[64] performed a study to asses hearing deficit in 20 individuals diagnosed with OSMF. hearing loss in individuals with grade I OSMF, there was a slight hearing loss in right and left side of the ears. Out of 9 Individuals 5 showed CHL whereas 4 out of 9 had mild CHL with grade II OSMF individuals and grade III OSMF individual showed bilateral mild CHL.A significant association was seen between grades of OSMF and hearing loss.

Sowbhagya et al (2016)[65], carried out a study to evaluate hearing loss in OSMF individuals on 40 individuals with OSMF and 20 normal individuals. All individuals had undergone audiometry and tympanometry test. In OSMF group 80 ears showed 44 (55%) ears in Type A curve, Type As in 13 (16.3%) ears, type Ad in 7 (8.8%) ears. And type B in 9 (11.3%) and type C in 7 (8.8%) ears whereas type A curve seen in all normal individuals. On pure tone audiometry (PTA) of study group Hearing was found to be normal in 47 (58%) ears, moderate hearing loss in 28 (35%) ears and mild hearing loss was found in 28 (35%) ears while hearing was normal in normal individuals. Author concluded that ET function may be affected in OSMF condition.

Alagiri Chandran (2016)[66], aimed to evaluate ET dysfunction with grade III and IV OSMF individuals. This study consisted of 30 cases with OSMF which included 15 stage IV (30 ears), 15 stage III (30 ears) and were compared with 15 normal controls and both groups were screened for tympanometry. In OSMF group Stage IV cases showed 76.3% positive audiogram, sclerosis of tympanic membrane seen in with 63.3% of cases and 43.3% of Stage III cases showed positive audiogram with 46.7% of cases having Sclerosis of tympanic membrane whereas negative audiogram was seen in normal individuals. The study concluded that ET function affect as disease progresses.

Kumar A (2018)[67] performed a study on 40 individuals with OSMF and 40 normal individuals, 80 ears in each group which were analysed for middle ear pressure by the use of impedance audiometry in OSMF Patients. The impedance audiometry test was performed and found statistically significant difference in middle ear pressure of OSMF patients and control. It has been concluded that the middle ear pressure got affected by disease process and cause hearing impairment.

ORAL SUBMUCOUS FIBROSIS AND TRACE ELEMENTS

Gupta et al (1987)[68] carried out a study to estimate the level of copper and zinc individuals with OSMF.40 individuals with OSMF and 10 normal individuals were included in the study. Atomic absorption spectrophotometer is used to measure the serum copper and zinc level. The result shows that there is significant rise in the copper level and decrease in zinc level in individuals with OSMF when compared to normal individuals and showed association between the trace elements level and occurrence of OSMF and other malignant condition.

According to Varghese et al (1987)[69] conducted a study on 200 individuals, 50 OSMF individuals, 50 with Oral leukoplakia and 50 individuals with oral cancer and 50 healthy subjects were selected for study. 5ml blood was taken and estimated for Cu and Zn level using AAS and Perkin- Elmer 400 AAS. There was significantly reduced the level of serum cu and Zn in individuals with OSMF when compared to cancer individuals. In OSMF individual's Cu/Zn ratio was increased. Hence to conclude that Cu/Zn ratio is a good biomarker for early oral cancer detection.

Kumar et al (1991)[70] selected 82 individuals of OSMF for assessment of therapeutic role of Zn alone or with either vitamin A or local cortisone in OSMF. 100 normal healthy individuals. For the treatment of grade I and II OSMF individuals oral Zinc therapy either alone or in combination with pharmacological doses of oral vitamin A proved to be significantly better. In grade III OSMF individuals on oral zinc in combination with local cortisone therapy proved to be significantly better than presently preferred local cortisone therapy. Hence, this study proves a beneficial role of oral zinc in therapy of OSMF.

Cunnigaiper D A et al (1995)71 undertook a study to evaluate trace elements and the hematological status with OSMF individuals. An increased platelet count and no significant change in the cell count, erythrocyte sedimentation rate and eosinophil count were also seen. In OSMF individuals a marked decrease in the levels of Fe, Hb%, ceruloplasmin, Zn and Cu and concluded that these trace elements were corelated with disease progression.

JR Hebert et al (2002)[72] assessed the dietary nutrients on oral precancerous lesions in a South Indian population. It comprised of precancerous lesions individuals and lesion free individuals with age and sex matched. A questionnaire was distributed for diet information for the both groups. 79% (485) women have precancerous lesions and 487 lesion free individuals. The most common form of tobacco use was reverse smoking among cases (81.9%) and controls (73.5%), and reverse smokers were 5.19 times more likely than chewers to have these lesions. Hence the study concluded that nutritional diet prevents the occurrence of precancerous lesion.

Luquman et al (2004)[73] performed a study on 15 patients with OSMF and 30 normal controls. 15 patients with OSMF were enrolled after diagnosis of clinical and histopathological Feature. Blood was collected from antecubital vein in antiseptic precaution from all the patients for estimation of the level of serum Cu and Fe level. Serum Cu level is 110.203micgm/dlt in OSMF patients and it is highly significant. Furthermore, serum Fe level is 80.287micgm/dlt and 86.33 micgm/dlt in OSMF and control group respectively. Serum cu level in OSMF showed increased value, and serum Fe level was reduced but it was not statistically significant.

Khanna and Karjodkar (2006)[74] evaluated the levels of trace elements (copper, iron and selenium) and circulating immune complexes in serum of OSMF, oral leukoplakia and oral squamous cell carcinoma (SCC) individuals. 37.5% polyethylene glycol used for estimation of Circulating immune complexes (CIC). Estimation of copper (Cu), selenium and iron were done using Colorimetric Dipyridyl, Oxylyl Dihydrazide and the Differential Pulse Cathodic Stripping Voltammetry method. There result showed that increased circulating immune complex levels in the cancer and precancerous individuals. The levels of Serum copper showed steady increase from precancerous to cancer individuals. On the other hand, levels of serum iron were significantly decreased in the cancer group whereas Selenium levels showed marked decrease in the cancer group. Hence to concluded that these are used as prognostic marker in cancer and precancer conditions

Nayak et al (2010)[75] analyzed the levels of trace elements in the population, who showed predominant use of areca nut on 20 cases of OSMF and 20 normal individuals. In this study the tissue and serum concentrations of Cu and Zn in 40 individuals was estimated by colorimeter method.

Savitha S Shettar et al (2010)[76] conducted a study on individuals with OSMF for that estimation of levels of zinc, copper and copper/zinc ratio in serum. A study consisted of 30 OSMF individuals and 30 normal individuals. Diagnosis was based on clinical and histopathology findings of OSMF. All Serum samples were estimated using semi-auto analyzer. In OSMF the mean serum levels of Zn and Cu were decreased when compared to normal individuals. Cu/Zn ratio and levels of Cu were increased in OSMF individuals compared to normal individuals. The mean serum levels of zinc showed no change through clinical and histological stages of OSMF. Cu/Zn ratio and levels of Cu revealed a gradual increase from grade I to IV individuals with OSMF. Cu and Zn may be used as prognostic markers of progression of OSMF.

Balpande A et al (2010)[77] conducted a study on individuals with OSMF, OL and OSCC for estimation of Cu/ Zn ratio, Cu, and Zn in serum. Serum samples was analyzed by colorimetric method using semi-automated analyzer. There was significantly decreased iron level and Cu/Zn ratio in OL, OSMF, and OSCC individuals. There was statistically significant difference of trace elements was found when compared the groups. These supplementary tests can be used in precancerous and cancer individuals for diagnosis and prognosis of the disease.

Ray et al (2011)[78] a study done on 60 individuals with oral leukoplakia and OSMF individuals. Venous blood was collected from 60 individuals for analysis with EDXRF technique. Out of the 16 detected elements (K, Si, Ca, V, Cr, Ni, Mn, Fe, Cu, Zn, Se, Br, Rb, Sr, Co, and Pb), Mn, Fe, Zn, Br, and Co showed remarkable alteration in their profile in both leukoplakia and OSMF individuals with respect to the normal healthy individuals. Zn, Br, and Fe showed gross depletion in both the group. There was inverse pattern in alternating concentrations of Mn and Co when compared to the control individuals.

Ganapathy et al (2011)[79] estimated the serum Fe levels and hemoglobin in individuals with OSMF and normal healthy individuals. A study group included 20 individuals, clinically diagnosed with OSMF with no other systemic history. 10 normal individuals and Iron deficiency anemia group consisted of 10 individuals. All the participants were subjected for estimation of hemoglobin and serum iron levels by using Sahli's method and Ferrene method. Hemoglobin and the serum iron level and hemoglobin were decreased in individuals with oral submucous fibrosis when compared with normal individuals.

Tadakamadla J et al (2011)[80] carried out a study to compare the levels of iron and copper in serum on 50 normal individuals and 50 individuals diagnosed with OSMF. The serum sample was analyzed by AAS. In OSMF Group there was increased level of copper and decreased level of iron when compared to normal individual. Author concluded that the copper level increased as the diseased progressed.

Ayinamudu et al (2012)[81] conducted a study on the level's Cu/Zn ratio, Cu and Zn in individuals with premalignant and malignant lesions in saliva. A study comprised of 10 individuals with SCC, 5 individuals with OSMF and 5 with oral leukoplakia. The sample of saliva was analyzed with inductive coupled mass spectrometry. When the data was compared between study and control group, there was statistically significant difference between levels of salivary zinc copper in SCC and Oral Leukoplakia and OSMF. Cu levels was high in OSMF individuals, whereas ratio of Cu/Zn decreased in OSMF individual. Saliva can be used as a diagnostic tool in premalignant and malignant lesions.

According to Shetty et al (2012)[82] a study aimed was to evaluate ascorbic acid levels and Fe in individuals with OSMF and without OSMF. Blood and saliva sample were collected and analyzed by dintrophenyl hydrazine and dipyridyle method. The serum and salivary ascorbic level and Fe level were reduced as the grading of OSMF. Iron and the ascorbic acid level can be used as diagnostic and prognostic tool of OSMF.

Hegde et al. (2012)[83] estimated and compared the hemoglobin and serum iron levels among individuals with OSMF and healthy individuals. A hospital-based study conducted on 30 OSMF individuals and 15 normal individuals. Blood sample was collected from all the participant and analyzed by Sahli's and Ferrene's methods. The result showed low levels of Fe and hemoglobin level when compared to normal individuals. And concluded that the estimation of these levels in OSMF disease can be helped in diagnosis, treatment and prevention of progression of OSMF.

Kamath et al (2013)[84] A systematic review conducted on biochemical markers in OSMF and demonstrated that most of the study showed cause and effect of areca nut in the progression of disease. Altered biomarkers in tissue and serum gives the exact pathogenesis and progression of the disease.

Shetty (2013)[85] A study conducted on individuals with OSMF, OSCC and Oral leukoplakia. Blood was collected from all the participants for the estimation of Cu, Fe and Zn. The levels of serum Cu was highly increased in OSMF individual when compared normal individuals. Decreased Zn level in serum in OSMF, OSCC and oral leukoplakia when compared to normal individuals. There was highly significant decreased level of Fe in OSMF. Cu/Zn ratio increased in OSMF, OSCC, and oral leukoplakia. A study concluded Cu/Zn ratio, Cu and Zn levels in serum may be used as a biomarker in precancerous and cancer lesion.

Kapoor S et al (2013)[86] determined the level of serum copper, zinc, iron and hemoglobin in clinically diagnosed cases of OSMF. 50 cases of OSMF compared with 50 controls. The serum copper, zinc, iron and hemoglobin of the individuals were measured by atomic absorption spectrometry, RANDOX kit and Sahli's method. A significant low-level serum zinc, iron and hemoglobin were observed in OSMF as compared to healthy control, whereas high level of serum copper was noted in cases of OSMF. The mean copper and Zinc ratio of control group 1.269 and OSMF group is 790, which was found to be much higher. Author concluded that these biological markers can be used for early detection of the diseased as well as its management.

Kode et al (2013)[87], The study aimed to evaluate the Cu, Zn And Mg levels in individuals with or without OSMF. Blood and saliva were collected for estimation of Cu Zn and Mg using differential pulse anodic stripping voltmeter and AAS and result showed the significant difference in levels of Zn and Fe in serum and in saliva Mg level was found highly significant in OSMF and without OSMF and ghutka habit individuals. So, susceptibility of cancer was seen in OSMF patients, as altered Serum Zn and Zn/Cu ratio was found in OSMF and is considered as the good biomarker.

Neethi H et al (2013)[88], carried out a study for the estimation and comparison of Cu and Zn levels in OSMF individuals. A study comprised 30 healthy and 30 histopathological diagnosed OSMF. Using the AAS the serum Cu and Zn level were estimated. And the result found higher level of Cu and Low levels of Zn in individual with OSMF. So, from these finding the role of Zn and Fe in the etiopathogenesis of OSMF was concluded.

S Khanna et al (2013)[89], conducted a study comprising of 90 individuals in which 30 individuals with OSMF, 30 individuals with OSCC and 30 normal individual. Blood sample was collected from all the participant and analyzed for Cu, Fe and Ng levels. Blood samples were estimated by graphite furnace AAS. The levels of Cu was increased in OSMF and OSCC group when compared to normal healthy individuals. Zn levels was slightly increased with OSMF and OSCC though it was not statistically significant. Cu, Zn Se and Mg levels are important in oral cancer.

Hosthor et al (2014)[90] conducted a study on patients with OSMF and OSCC for evaluation of Cu, Fe, Mg Zn and Ca levels in serum. Serum samples were collected from all the participant and analyzed by Electronic absorption calorimetric method. Fe, Zn and Mg levels were decreased in both the groups whereas, the Ca level was increased in Cancer group. Author concluded that copper is the main predictor amongst the all other tested trace elements.

Guruprasad R et al (2014)[91], conducted a study to evaluate Vit C level and Fe with individual with OSMF comparing with the healthy individual study comprised of 35 OSMF and 50 healthy patients. Venous blood was collected. Vitamin C level was obtained using dinitroplynyl hydrazine method and Ramsey's method was used to estimate the iron level. Vitamin C and iron level in serum was reduced with OSMF individuals 0.4±0.23mg/dl and 98.87±18μg/dl respectively. From the study it can be concluded that the deficiency of iron and vitamin C level with the habit of chewing areca nut act as the confounding factor in OSMF disease.

F Mohammad et al (2015)[92] performed a study on 60 patients, out of which 30 were with OSMF and 30 healthy individuals. Unstimulated whole saliva was collected from each patient, saliva Cu level was estimated using calorimetric method. Commercially available areconoid product which was used by the pat and subjected to Cu analysis through AAS method. Biopsy was performed on OSMF patients for histopathological estimation. There was negative correlation of Cu content with 3 different arecanoid products and different histological grades of OSMF. There was progressive increase level of salivary Cu in OSMF patients when compared with healthy patients.

In a study by Shetty et al in (2015)[93],200 individuals divided into group 1 and group 2. 50 patients with oral leukoplakia, group2 were OSMF patients, group3 were 50OSCC and group4 were healthy ones. 5ml unstimulated saliva was collected from each patient and were centrifuged. The level of Cu, and Zn were compared using GBV Avanta atom absorption spectrophotometer.

Hameed et al (2015)[94] evaluated 89 patients in each group who diagnosed with OSMF and healthy patients. Serum samples were analyzed by calorimetric method using semiauto analyzer and the difference in the result were noted. In OSMF individual Fe level was decreased when compared to normal individual. For the diagnosis and prognosis of OSMF serum Fe should be a part of routine assessment.

Saurabh et al (2015)[95] in a study of 60 individuals with OSMF and 30 normal individuals. Blood sample was collected from all the participant for estimation of Fe and protein level. The result showed that when compared to normal individuals there was statistically significant reduction of serum iron and increased levels of protein.

Yadav et al (2015)96 conducted a study on fifty individuals with clinically diagnosed OSMF fibrosis and fifty controls. The level of serum zinc was significantly lesser among cases (73.48 ± 24.21) compared with controls (119.48 ± 52.78). However, the serum copper level was significantly higher among cases (155.50 ± 40.13) than controls (100.40 ± 24.52). The level of serum iron was lower among the cases (66.57± 27.76) as compared to controls (94.19 ± 35.70), and the difference was statistically significant.

Srilekha. M (2015)[97] investigated the Cu, Zn and Cu/Zn ratio in serum in individuals with OSMF and normal individuals. It comprised of total 50 individuals, 25 with OSMF and 25 normal individuals. 5 ml blood was collected from all the participants and analyzed by spectrophotometric method. The result showed that serum copper level was increased whereas serum Zn level was found to be decreased. A study concluded deficiency of Zn and high level of Cu seen in OSMF individual.

According to Okade et al (2015)[98], in an investigation of trace elements involving 60 individuals equally divided into two groups containing OSMF patients in which 5ml of saliva were collected and the estimated for trace elements level using AAS using Wet Ashi method.

Mean salivary Zn and iron level and Cu/Zn ratio were found to be decreased. Mean Cu levels were increased in OSFM when compared to the controls and concluded that it can be used in early detection and treatment of OSMF.

Tiwari R et al (2016)[99] conducted a study on 40 patients with PMD and oral cancer and 30 normal patients. Blood samples were collected from all the participants for estimation of Cu, Zn and CIC. Samples were analyzed by spectrophotometric and colorimetric methods. The highest level of CIC was found in oral cancer, PMD individuals and low levels in normal individuals. In Oral cancer Cu level was high followed by PMD individuals when compared to normal individuals. Decreased level of Fe was found in PMD individuals and those with oral cancer when compared to normal individuals.

D Bhardwaj et al (2016)[100], performed a study to assess association between Fe levels and Hb in individuals with OSMF. A study comprised of 120 individuals, 40 subjects with OSMF 40 with IDA with tobacco chewing habit, 40 healthy. Blood was collected from each participant for estimation of levels of Fe and Hb. Samples were analyzed by using Ferrozine method and sahalyl's method. There was statistically significant difference found in three groups. There is the reduction in serum Fe and Hb levels as the stage increases of OSMF.

Kallalli et al (2016)[101] performed a study to evaluate Fe levels with 30 OSMF individuals. For the estimation of tissue and serum Fe levels vitros 250 photometry was used. There was significant decrease level of serum and tissue Fe with OSMF individuals as compared to normal individuals.

H Kumar el at (2016)[102] investigated 70 individuals equally divided in OSMF and Healthy individuals. AAS was used to estimate the levels of serum Cu and Fe. The result showed significant increase in serum Cu level in OSMF individuals. Whereas serum Fe level decreases as clinical staging progress of OSMF and it was statically significant.

More C B et al (2016)[103] performed a study which aimed to estimate the level of trace elements in OSMF, OSCC and oral leukoplakia individuals. Total 30 individuals having oral submucous fibrosis, OSCC and oral leukoplakia included in the study. The incision or punch biopsy were performed in each individual, the level serum of Fe, Cu and Zn were estimated using calorimetric method with semiautomated analyzer. The result found increased serum Cu level in OSMF, OSCC and oral leukoplakia individual when compared to normal individual. Whereas the decreased level Zn and Fe was seen in OSMF, OSCC and oral leukoplakia individuals when compared with normal individuals.

M Thakur et al (2017)[104] Schwartz (1952) in a study of 80 patients histologically and clinically staged into OSMF group, TIBC and serum Ferritin level were estimated using tulip iron and TIBC kit and bios microwell ELISA diagnostic system kit. From the result it has been found that the Hb, serum iron and serum Ferritin levels were reduced in OSMF patients and TIBC was increased as compared with controls.

S Latoo et al (2017)[105] conducted a study on 30 individuals with OSMF and 30 normal individuals. Blood samples were analysed for serum the levels of Fe and Cu by AAS. There was high Cu and low levels of Fe in individuals with OSMF when compared to normal individuals. Hence the study concluded that as the stages of OSMF increases, Cu level also increase.

Y V Jani et al in 2017[106]. The sample consisted of 150 individuals, out of which the cases group consisting of 100 OSMF individuals and control group consisting of 50 individuals. All the cases were established of having OSMF by histopathological examination. The blood sample was collected from all 150 individuals and evaluated by digital autoanalyzer photometer for serum level of copper and iron by the colorimetric method. The mean serum copper level increases while the mean serum iron level decreases with the progression in the severity of clinical and histological stages of OSMF.

Bhalerao S et al (2018)[107] Total 66 patients were selected for the study out of which 22 OSMF, 22 individuals without OSMF with areca nut chewing habit and 22 normal individuals. 5ml of venous blood sample was taken and estimated for iron level usingby Ferrozine method. In OSMF there was decreased level of Fe and vit C in serum and saliva when compared to normal individuals. Therefore, regular monitoring of betel nut habitual should also be carried out because they are at higher risk of developing OSMF in future. Study indicates that saliva also can be used as a diagnostic biomarker in OSMF disease. Estimation of iron and vitamin C in OSMF individuals would help in management, in developing therapies based on the trace element expression.

CLINICAL EXAMINATION OF OSMF

In OSMF individuals thorough clinical examination and complete history was taken for each individual in the OPD of Department of Periodontology and Department of Ear Nose and Throat. The OSMF individual were recruited according to the clinical staging of Khanna's classification. Vernier Calliper was used to measure the interincisal distance between the maxillary and mandibular central incisors edges and maximum mouth opening. (fig 1&2)

Classification of OSMF:

Stage I: Common symptoms like acute ulceration, recurrent stomatitis burning sensation with normal mouth opening.[108]

Stage II: Mottled and marble like sheet appearance of buccal mucosa which is fibrous on palpation associated with 26- 35 mm of interincisal distance of maxillary and mandibular teeth.[108]

Stage III: Pale firmly attached to underlying tissues of buccal mucosa, trismus atrophy of vermilion border, vertical fibrous bands seen on soft palate, anterior faucial pillars and pterygomandibular raphe associated with 15- 25 mm of inter incisal distance.[108]

Physical examination:

A general physical examination was carried out to look for any gross debilitating condition. Following information was recorded in history and a detailed intraoral examination was carried out and recorded for each patient.

a. Prominent symptoms such as painful ulcerations, burning sensation of mouth, inability to blow cheek, intolerance to hot and spicy food.

b. Unable to swallow or excessive salivation or referred pain in the ears.

c. Site of involvement - Buccal mucosa, retro molar region, anterior pillar, uvula, soft/ hard palate, lips. Clinical signs such as blanching, ulcerations and vesicle formations were also noted.

d. Presence and distribution of fibrous bands - Distribution and direction of fibrous bands were checked. Bilateral palpation was done by placing the finger posteriorly in the retro molar area, anteriorly over the buccal mucosa and finally-palpating the labial mucosa.

e. Inter-incisal mouth opening - The distance between the edges of maxillary and mandibular central incisors was measured in millimeter.

f. History was taken regarding any change in hearing efficiency. The pure tone audiometry was done for all the individual

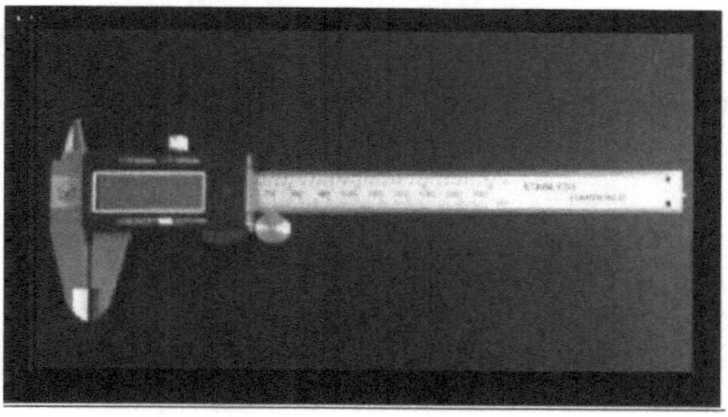

Figure 4: Vernier calliper

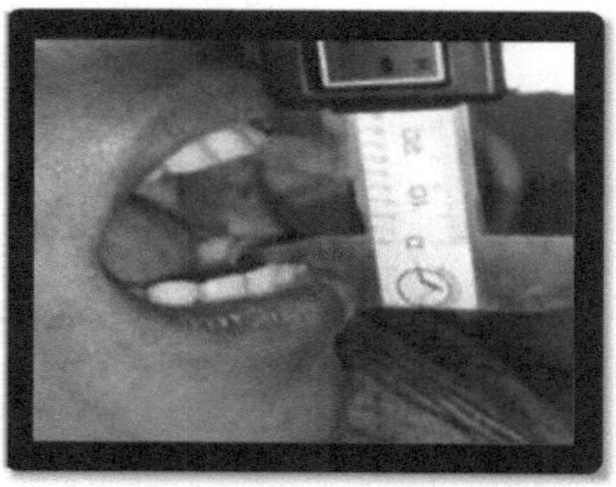

Figure 5: Interincisal measurement using Vernier calliper

The colour of oral mucosa was assessed in natural light and scored as: normal pink (0), red or deep pink (1), pale white (2) and blanched white (3).

The fibrous bands were palpated and scored as follows: No fibrous bands (0), one or two solitary fibrous bands (1), bands felt nearly in the entire surface (2), adherent fibrous band producing binding and rigidity of mucosa (3).

The individuals were enquired about burning sensation while taking spicy food, pan, tobacco, hot beverages, etc. and scored as: no burning sensation (0), mild (l), moderate (2) and severe (3).

PROCEDURE FOR SERUM EVALUATION OF TRACE ELEMENTS

Serum separation

5 ml venous blood was collected & stored at 37 degree Celsius for 1 hour followed by centrifugation at 3000rpm for 6 min. Separated serum was stored in a plain sterile glass bulb at 4 degree Celsius & estimation of trace elements Cu, Zn and Fe was done by atomic absorption spectrophotometry.

Atomic Absorption Spectrophotometry[109.110,111]

The process of atomic absorption spectrophotometry has been explained schematically in the figure below.

Atomic Absorption Process

The ground state atom absorbs specific wavelength light energy as it enters the excited state. The number of atoms in the light pathway increases with the increase in amount of light. By measuring the amount of light absorbed, a quantitative determination of the amount of analyte can be made. The specific determination of individual elements can be done by using the specific light sources and careful selection of wavelength.

The basic difference between atomic emission and atomic absorption is as follows:

In atomic emission, the flame serves a dual purpose: It converts the sample aerosol into an atomic vapor and then thermally elevates the atom to excite state. When return to ground state these atoms emit light which is detected by the instrument. The intensity of light emitted is related to concentration of the element of interest in solution.

Converting the sample aerosol into atomic vapor, which then absorb light from primary source (hollow cathode lamp or electrodeless discharge lamp) is the only function of flame in atomic absorption.

Five basic components of atomic absorption as follows:

1. The light source which emits the spectrum of the element of interest.

2. An —absorption celll where the sample atoms are produced (lamp, graphite furnace, MHS cell, FIAS cell, FIMS cell)

3. A monochromator is used for light dispersion.

4. A detector, which measures the light intensity and amplifies the signal

5. A display to show the reading after it has been processed by electronic instrument

Atomic absorption instruments have two types: Single beam and double beam

The light source (hallow cathode lamp or electrodeless discharge lamp) emits specific spectrum to element, which is focused through sample cell into monochromator.

To differentiate between the light source and the emission from sample cell, the light source must be electronically modulated or mechanically chopped.

The monochromator disperses the light of specific wavelength and isolated passes through detector, which is a photomultiplier tube. Depending upon the light intensity an electric current is produced and processed by the electronic instrument.

The amount of light attenuation in the sample cell can be measured by electronic device which gives the actual sample concentration. With single -beam system, a short warm up period is required to allow the sample lamp to stabilize.

Sample preparation for copper and zinc:

To determine copper in serum, the serum sample was diluted with an equal volume of deionized water. And for zinc detection, sample is diluted in 1:5 with deionized water.

Analysis:

The Cu (copper) and Zn (zinc) concentration were determined and listed using the —standard condition‖ section

By diluting the Cu stock standard solution, the Cu standards were prepared., described in "Standard Conditions" for copper, with 10%(v/v) glycerol. A 10% (v/v) was used as a blank solution when determining copper.

For zinc, the stock standard was diluted with 5% (v/v) glycerol and the zinc standards were prepared. A 5 % (v/v) blank glycerol solution was used for zinc determination.

Sample Preparation for Iron

In a polyethylene tube, serum sample (1.0 mL) was diluted with equal volume of 20%(w/v) TCA solution. Sample preparation for iron the tube was capped loosely and the serum sample was mixed and then heated in a heating block for 15 min at 900

C. The tube was cooled and then centrifuged.

Analysis: -

The conditions which are listed in the standard condition section were used to analyse the supernatant in iron determination. By diluting the iron stock solution appropriate iron standards were prepared, described in the —standard section‖ for iron with 10% (w/v) TCA.

A 10% (w/v) TCA solution should be used for the blank. Since the sample were diluted 1:2 with TCA, the instrument was calibrated to read 2 × the actual standards concentration, so as to read concentration directly.

Standard Operating Procedure for Flame Technique

The burner was aligned and feeded blank to make zero. Optimize signal command was clicked for blank 0.000. The standard was then feeded according to cook book to observe the absorbance. And the analysis was started by clicking on START.

1 Switch ON PC. Switch ON The instrument.

2. Open _Spectra AA‘ Software

3. Click on Work sheet

4. Create new worksheet by giving specific name. If already exist, then select that one.

5. Give the method name.

6. Then select the required element.

7. Now element is added, Double click on that element for editing the method. In Method tab Select Manual and Absorption for flame. Flame type default one for Flame technique. Save IT.

8. In sequence tab enter the sample name.

9. Go to analysis mode. Click on Optimization align the lamp to get minimum lamp gain.

10. Once you start it will ask for Blank and standards after that ask for samples.

11. After Analysis is done go to Report. Select the required worksheet and take the print.

PROCEDURE FOR PURE TONE AUDIOMETRY21

Audiological assessment was carried out in the Department of Audiology and Speech therapy. For all the individual‘s PTA was performed by ELKON Advanced Digital Audiometer in sound proof room. Individuals with OSMF and without OSMF were undergone for PTA to analyze BC and AC threshold for tones from 250, 500,1000,2000, and 4000 Hz. If the intensity was raised above the normal level it measures the degree of hearing impairment at that frequency.

Depending upon AC-BC gap values, hearing impairment was quantitatively graded.

Interpretation of audiogram

The hearing threshold level are 250,500,1000,2000 and 4000 Hz only. The deafness can be categorised by air conduction is as follows:[21]

1. 10-15 dB- Normal hearing
2. 16-25 dB-Minimal HL
3. 26-40 dB- Mild HL
4. 41-55 dB-Moderate HL
5. 56-70 dB –Moderate to severe HL
6. 71-90 dB-Severe HL
7. Above 90 is profound deafness

At the time of PTA if there is hearing deficit the next step is to examine whether there is sensory or mechanical problem (sensorineural or conductive Hearing loss). The bone vibrator was used for the distinction between AC and BC which bypass the mechanical parts of the middle ear. In conductive Hearing Loss there is better hearing on use of bone than air. All the participants undergone for both AC and BC by PTA and plotted the graph. The mean values of AC and BC was recorded for each individual.

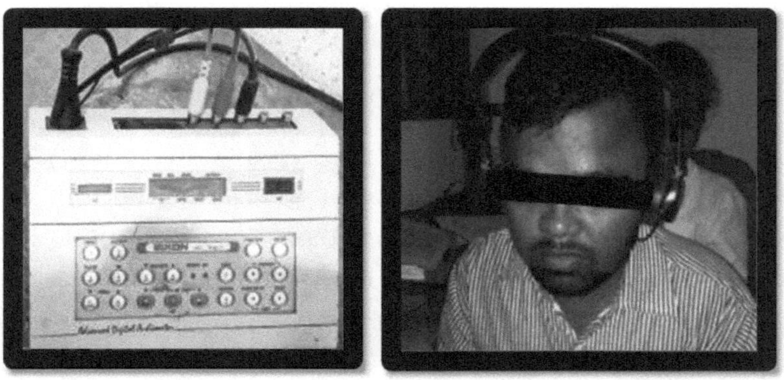

Figure 6: Pure Tone Audiometry

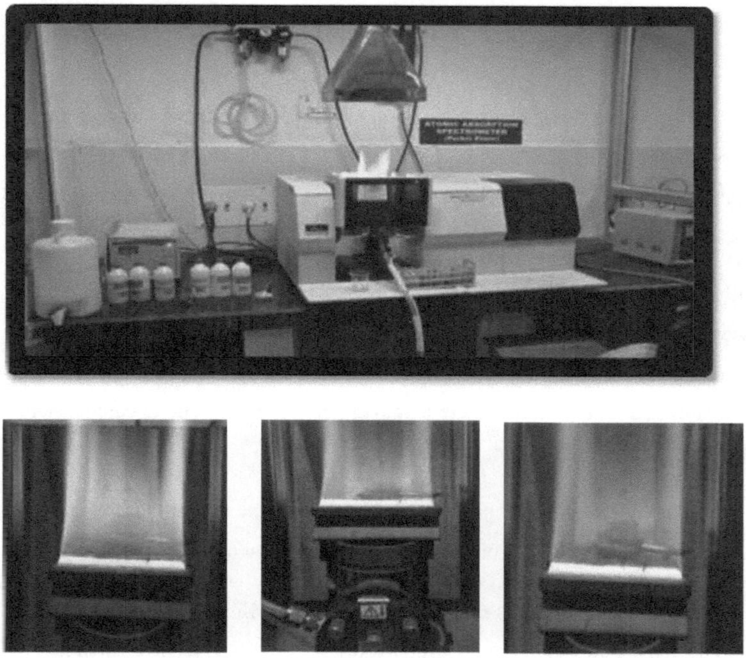

Copper **Iron** **Zinc**

Figure 7: Atomic absorption spectrophotometry

DISCUSSION

OSMF is a slowly progressive disease affecting oral mucosa of the oral cavity of leading to fibrosis of oral mucous membrane causing restriction of jaw and tongue movements resulting in inability to eat and deglutition.[60]

According to SM Haider, OSMF starts at fauces or posterior part of oral cavity. As severity increases it progresses to involve oral mucosa of anterior part. Similar findings were found in our study.[112]

OSMF is slowly progressive disease in which fibrous bands are formed in the oral mucosa leading to severe restriction of tongue movements. Various authors have reported degenerative changes in the muscles of soft palate, edema, and atrophy of the palatal and paratubal muscle.[59,113]

Physiologically opening and closing of ET is important. This ET is connected to middle ear cavity by nasopharynx. However, on normal opening of ET, the atmospheric pressure is equalized in middle ear whereas the closing of ET protects the middle ear from unwanted pressure fluctuations and loud sound. If there is impairment in closing and opening function of ET leads to hearing disability due to the middle ear.[21]

The muscles which are attached to soft palate is tensor veli palatine and levetor veli palatine. A study conducted by Binnie and Cowson have stated degeneration of muscle fibres.[114]

Some of the authors conducted studies on individuals with OSMF , observed tissues under microscope and demonstrated that dense collagen bundles that are oriented and extended into underlying muscle.[115] Rajendra et al reported extensive fatty infiltration between bundle of muscles , focal lysis and hypercontraction of myofibers of OSMF patients.[116] Dysfunction and patency of ET due to involvement of surrounding muscles caused a discomfort in ear leading to mild to moderate hearing loss with OSMF disease.[116]

There is numerous hearing sensitivity test are available for measuring hearing sensitivity test, in this study Pure tone audiometry was used.

In conductive hearing loss, normal bone conduction threshold and air conduction threshold decrease than normal threshold. It is abnormality of outer and middle ear. It affects air conduction but bone conduction signals that does not pass through the outer or middle ear.[65]

The rate of distribution of precancerous and cancerous conditions is very high. In recent years prevalence of precancerous lesion was much higher than cancer lesions. At present detection of established carcinoma and progression of disease from pre-malignant to malignant relies heavily on histopathological examination. Thus, it is necessary for reliable and sensitive biochemical test. It can be used for diagnosis of disease at early stage.

Recently much emphasis has been given towards detection of trace elements in oral cancer and precancerous condition because of the encouraging result of the studies on head and neck carcinoma, lymphoma, lung carcinoma and breast carcinoma. Abdulla et al. detected Zinc and copper levels were in head and neck carcinoma for the first and found that in whole blood plasma the level of zinc was significant depressed and level of Cu/Zn ratio was and elevated. Author concluded the levels cu and Zn may be used for prognosis in cancer of head and neck[33,35]

Though review of literature reveals very few studies conducted to find out eustachian tube dysfunction and trace elements leading to hearing impairment in OSMF, it does not show a comprehensive study. Hence a study conducted to evaluate and compare the levels of Cu, Zn and Fe and eustachian tube dysfunction leading to hearing impairment in OSMF. So, it was thought worthwhile to undertake the present study to evaluate and compare the Eustachian tube dysfunction leading to hearing impairment & levels of trace elements in serum in individuals with and without OSMF.

Trivedy et al have stated chewing areca nut releases Cu into the saliva as areca nut have high Cu content a high content of Cu in areca nut and concluded elevated levels of Cu in tissue sample of OSMF in comparison to normal mucosa.[14]

Shrilekha et al (2015) A study conducted on 30 individuals in test group and 30 individuals in control group for estimation of copper, copper zinc ratio and zincin serum. She concluded a significant high level of Cu and low level of Zn in OSMF individuals than the control group.[97]

Luquman et al (2004) conducted a study in 15 patients with OSMF within the age range 17-40 years and 30 normal controls within the same range to estimate the level of serum Cu and Fe level. Serum Cu level was 110.203micgm/dlt in OSMF.

Various authors reported that the Copper can upregulate the expression of enzyme lysloxidase in the oral mucosa leading to fibrosis. It may be due to Cu stabilizes the enzyme activity by increasing its half-life and also at the molecular level the N-terminus of Exon-1 of lysyl oxidase molecule has copper binding site and this interaction may up regulate the expression of the enzyme at cellular level. The elevated level of serum Cu in patients with OSMF could cause upregulation of lysyl oxidase enzyme for crosslinking of collagen and elastin.[15,74,80]

Previous researchers observed high levels of Cu in tissue as well as in serum in premalignant and malignant conditions. In the contrary Trivedy reported Cu level normal in serum with OSMF individuals. Reason behind High levels of Cu in serum with premalignant and malignant conditions was not known. This might be due to more production of ceruloplasmin by liver. It is an inflammatory response.[76,80,101]

Zinc plays the role of an antioxidant in prevention of carcinogenesis by two mechanisms:

One is the protection of sulfahydral groups against oxidation and the inhibition of the protection of reactive oxygen species production by transition metals. Secondly, supra physiological concentration of Zn has antioxidants like effect in organelle-based systems and isolated cell-based systems. Thus, the decrease in Zn levels and Zn dependent SOD is said to be an indicator of early mucosal changes preceding carcinogenesis.[82]

Zinc deficiency causes (COX 2) upregulation of cyclooxygenase. There is an over expression of COX -2 enhances proliferation of cell, inhibits apoptosis, modulates angiogenesis and there by contributing to carcinogenesis. (Barch 1986) reported Zn plays a role in maintain the integrity of membrane. It also intricates in the stability of membrane and lipid peroxidation. Zinc plays a role in RNA, DNA polymerase and its activation effect on membrane bound adenyl cyclase, these suggest carcinogenesis role of zinc. Decreased level of Zn may lead to initiation of cancer through activation of NF-Kb resulting in initiation of tumor signaling.[90,117]

In OSMF Iron levels are reduced due to Decreased Fe level in OSMF might be due to more use of Iron in collagen synthesis leading to utilization of Fe in collagen synthesis, epithelial vascularity declined. It causes burning sensation, erosion and fibrosis.[79]

Serum Fe should be a part of routine assessment and should be used for diagnosis of disease.10 In hydroxylation of proline and lysine, Fe is required for collagen synthesis through enzyme. Peptyl proline hydroxylase needs molecular oxygen and ferrous ions co factors. Hence, in OSMF individual serum Fe level is decreased.[80,91,95,96,100,104,106]

Some of the studies have been conducted in relation to OSMF and hearing but the present study compared the trace elements level and hearing loss in patients with and without OSMF.

Detection of trace elements in OSMF can open the doors for novel analytic and therapeutic modalities in areas of medicine and oncology. Thus, Eustachian tube functions is affected in OSMF, hence individuals with OSMF should be screened for hearing loss.

SUMMARY AND CONCLUSION

With the objective of determining the correlation of OSMF and eustachian tube dysfunction leading to hearing impairment and the levels of trace elements in serum of the individuals with submucous fibrosis and hearing impairment.

Possible contribution and translator component

There are 600 million of people who chew betel quid throughout their life regularly. Betel quid chewing is major contributory factors of precancerous and cancer of oral cavity in India and many other countries.

OSMF is slowly progressive disease of oral mucous membrane and termed as premalignant lesion. Its prevalence in India is very high ranging from 0 to 0.2%. OSMF affects oral mucosa causing stiffness and rigidity leading to partial trismus.[2]

OSMF affects the ET function leading to hearing loss as it also affects other part of the oral cavity such as oral mucosa, soft and hard palate, pharynx and naso pharynx. There occurs a slow hearing deficit which can have functional and clinical significance. Thus, these patients show impaired responses to loud sounds, leading to conductive hearing loss.

OSMF have multifactorial etiology which includes ingestion of chilies, genetic, chewing areca nut, nutritional deficiency etc. the main ingredient of areca nut is arecadine, arecoline, guacine, guyacoline.[56,57]

OSMF is a precancerous in nature and its rate of transformation into malignancy is in the range of 7-13% and was first describe in 1956.[60]

OSMF have multifactorial etiology, further research is needed for to sensitive, specific and faster test. Biochemical and immunological alteration in serum of OSMF individuals can help for appropriate and early diagnosis and line of treatment. To find the levels of trace elements in OSMF opened the doors for newer diagnostic and therapeutic endeavors.

AAS is the reliable, most efficient and simple to use methods to detect the level of metals and metalloids in samples. The AAS method highly sensitive and excellent detection limit, wide linear dynamic multielement capability also have capabilities to measure isotopes ratios, high sample at relatively low cost. The level of trace elements is affected in hearing impairment in OSMF patient. The habit of chewing areca nut is common practice found in young individuals, so the number of young individuals affected by OSMF are also common. As the severity of disease is progress the involvement of Para tubal muscle is seen, which results in the hearing impairment in young individuals. For identification of hearing sensitivity pure tone audiometry is used and also gives degree and configuration of hearing loss and provides a proper diagnosis and management.

Identification of level of trace element in OSMF may help

1. To identify an individual at risk for malignant transformation.

2. The level of hearing loss can also be determined.

3. To determine prognosis, improve patient acceptance and optimize treatment outcome in individual.

4. To determine the disease severity.

Implication

OSMF is mostly diagnosed on the basis of clinico-histological evaluation. These methods have some limitation. These methods are easy to use but these parameters will not prove beneficial for the assessment of the severity of the disease and involvement of adjacent structure. Additional qualitative and quantitative methods or tools for determination of trace elements in serum. The hearing assessment for diagnosis of loss of hearing have also been determined for disease recognition and prediction.

Despite advancements made in the areas of OSMF diagnosis and prognosis, only limited studies have been conducted to identify trace element that predict disease progression prior to clinical and histological manifestations. Teenagers and youths are getting more attracted to commercially available areca nut products like Gutkha and so the prevalence of OSMF is more in younger generation and one of the adverse effects of OSMF on function of eustachian tube leading to hearing impairment. Previous studies demonstrated that loss of hearing reduces the quality of life. Randomized clinical trial using antioxidant like Zn and Fe can be designed and if found effective may provide for treatment of hearing impairment in CSMF individual.

BIBLIOGRAPHY

1. Murti PR, Bhonsale RB, Gupta PC et al. Etiology of Oral submucous fibrosis with special reference to the role of areca nut chewing. J Oral Pathol Med 1995.24;145-152.
2. Pindborg JJ, Sirsat SM. Oral submucous fibrosis. Oral Surg Oral Med Oral Pathol 1966;22(6):764-79.
3. Shafer WG, Hine MK, Levy BM et al. A textbook of oral pathology. Prism Book Pvt ltd 4th edition 1993.
4. Mehta FS, Hammer JE. Tobacco-related oral mucosal lesion and conditions in India. Jaypee Brother medical pub. Ltd. 1993.
5. Ranganathan K, Umadevi M, Joshua E et al. Oral submucous fibrosis: A case control study in Chennai, South India. J. Oral Pathol and Med 2004;33:274- 277.
6. Jayanthi V, Probert CSJ, Sher KS, Mayberry JF. Oral submucous fibrosis- a preventable disease. Gut 1992;33:4-6.
7. Murthi PR, Gupta PC, Bhosale RB et al. Effect on the incidence of oral submucous fibrosis intervention in the areca nu chewing habit. J Oral Pathil Med 1990;19:99-100.
8. Paisaat DK. Oral submucous fibrosis. Int. J Oral Surg 1981;10:307312.
9. Sinor PN, Gupta PC, Murti PR. A case control study of oral submucous fibrosis with special reference to the etiologic role of areca nut. J. Oral Pathol and Med 1990;19:94-98.
10. Canniff JP, Harvey W. The aetiology of oral submucous fibrosis the stimulation of collagen synthesis by extract of areca nut. Int. J Oral Surg 1981;10: 165-167.
11. Tsai CH, Chou MY, Chang YC. The up-regulation of cyclooxygenase-2 expression in human buccal mucosal fibroblast by arecoline: a possible role in the pathogenesis of oral submucous fibrosis. J Oral Pathol Med 2003 ; 32:146- 153.
12. Jeng JH, Kuo ML, Hanh LJ et al. Genotoxi and non genotoxic effect of betel quid ingredients on oral mucosal fibroblast invitro. J Dent Res, May 1994;73(5):1043-1049.

13. Seedat HA, Vanwyk CW. Submucous fibrosis in ex-betel nut chewer: a report of 14 cases. J oral pathol, 1988; 17:226-229.

14. Trivedy C et al. Copper content in areca catechu (betelnut) products and oral submucous fibrosis. Lancet 1997;340:1447.

15. Trivedy C, Warnakulsuriya KAAS, Hazarey VK et al. The upregulation of lysy; oxidase in oral submucous fibrosis and squamous cell carcimona. J Oral Pathol Med 199;28:246-251.

16. Gupta PC, Warnakulasuita S. Global epidemiology of areca nut usage. Addict Biol 2002;7:77-83.

17. Sirsat SM, Khanolkar VR. Submucous fibrosis of the palate in diet-preconditioned Wistar rats. Induction by local painting of capsaicin—an optical and electron microscopic study. Arch Pathol. 1960 Aug;70:171-9.

18. Ramanathan K. Oral Pre-cancer condition in peninsular Malaysia. Med J Malaysia 1979;33(3);216-221.

19. Rajendra R, Suganthan CK, Remani P, Ankathi IR et al. Cell mediated humoral immune responses in oral subuvous fibrosis. Cancer 1986;58:2628- 2631.

20. Varghese I, et al. Prevalence of OSMF among the cashew workers of Kerala, South India J of Cancer 1986;23:101-04

21. Chaudhary MS, Mohite DP, Gupta R, Patil S, Gosavi S, et al. Evaluation of Hearing Efficiency in Patients with Oral Sub mucous Fibrosis. Otolaryngology 2013;3(4):143

22. PL Dhingra, Shruti Dhingra. Textbook of diseases of ear nose and throat, 6thedi. Elsevier A division of reed Elsevier India Pvt Ltd.

23. Brown CJ, Chenery S,R,N. Snith B, Mason C, Tomkins A, Robert GJ. Environmental influences on the trace element content off teeth: implication for disease and nutritional status. Arch. Oral Biol 2004;49(9):705-717.

24. Shanker AK, Mode of action and toxicity of trace element, Trace Elements: Nutritional Benefits. Environmental Contamination and Health Implication, CRIDA Hyderabad 2008:523-553.

25. White DK, Miller AS, Gomez L. Occurrence of oral squamous cell carcinoma in Person under 50 years of Age. J Am Dent Asso 1976;92:573.

26. Sood RK, Ghooi AM, Bhambhai H. Serum copper studies in malignancies. Ind. J. Surg 1976;38:303-308.

27. Clark J,Gubler. Copper metabolism in man. J A m Med Asso 1956;161:530- 534.

28. Harper HA, Rodwell VW, Meyers PA. Water and Mineral metabolism, 574 from Review of Physiology and chemistry. Lange Medical Publications, Los Atlas California 1977.
29. Jha JM. Serum copper/zinc ratio in oral malignancy. Ind. J Med. Res.1985;81(6):602-606.
30. Mcquity JT, DeWys WD, Monaco L, Strain WH, Rob CG. Inhibition of tumor growth by dietry zinc deficiency. Cancer Res 1970;30:1381-1390.
31. Waren BC, Evenson MA. Determination of zinc and copper in Serum. Clinic Chem 1975;21:619.
32. Burtis CA, Ashwood ER. Tietz textbook of chemistry, 3rd ed. Philadelphia: WB Saunders, 1999:531-2.
33. Schwartz MK. Role of trace elements in cancer. Cancer Res 1975;35:3481- 3487.
34. Batsaki JG. Tumors of the head and neck, Clinical and Pathological consideration; William and Wilkins Baltimore/London 1979.
35. Abdulla M, Biorklund A, Mathur A, Wallenius K. Zinc and copper levels in whole blood and plasma from patients with squamous cell carcinoma of the head and neck. J Surg Oncol 1979;12:107-113.
36. Bhardwaj VP, Luthra VK. Acid Phosphatase and DNA Studies in DMBA-induced experimental oral carcinogenesis in hamaster cheek pounch. Ind J. Med. Res 59.401-412.
37. Brieter DN, Diasio RB, Neifeld JP, Roush ML, Rosenberg SA. Serum copper and zinc measurement in patients with osteogenic sarcoma. Cancer 1978;42:498-602.
38. Chakravarthy PK. Zinc in human malignancies. Neoplasma 1986;33(1).85-90.
39. Derise NL, Ritchey SJ. Mineral composition of normal humans enamel and dentine and the relation of compositions to dental caries:II Microminerals 1974. J. Dent. Res;53(4):853-858.
40. Brudevold F, Stedman LT, Spinnelli MA, Amdur BH, Gross P. Study of zinc in human teeth. Oral Biol 1963;8:135-144.
41. Wallenius K, Mathur A, Abdulla M. Assessment of sub- clinical ainc deficiency for carcinogenetic and other long term studies in rats. Arch. Oral Biol 1978:23(12):1077-82.
42. Miles DA. Functions of zinc : A Literature Resume, J. Oral Med, 1982 (37): 93-97.

43. Burket LW. Oral Medicine : Diagnosis and Treatment, 8thed. Philadelphia, J.B. Lippincott Company, 1984.
44. Dennes E, Tupper T, WormallA.The zinc content of Erythrocytes and Leukocutes of Blood from normal and Leukemic Subjects. Biochem.J. 1961: (78);578-587.
45. DaviesJ, Musa M, Dormandy T. Measurement of Plasma Zinc II. Malignant Disease, J. Clin,Pathol, 1968(21):363-365.
46. Good R. A., West A., Day N. K., Dong Z. W., Fernandes G. Effects of undernutrition of host cell and organ function. Cancer Research. 1982;42:737s–746s.
47. Todd. Clinical diagnosis and management by laboratory method:188-193.
48. Vasudevan DM. Textbook of biochemistry. Jaypee Brothers, medical publisher Ltd. 1st ed. 1996.
49. Andrews NC. Disorder of iron metabolism. N. Engl J Med, 2000;342(5):364.
50. Chatterjea MV, ,Shinde R. Textbook of biochemistry. Jaypee brother 5th ed. 2002: 534-545.
51. Tietz NW. Fundamentals of clinical chemistry 3rd ed. 818-824.
52. Talwar GP, Shrivastava LM, Mondgil KD. Textbook of biochemistry and human biology. Prentice- hall of India Pvt Ltd. 2nd ed. 1989:551-560.
53. Deb AC. Fundamentals of biochemistry. New central book agency Pvt. Ltd. 4th ed. 1994:442-453.
54. Deb AC. Fundamentals of biochemistry. New central book agency Pvt. Ltd.8th ed. 2002:424-448.
55. Afroz N, Hasan SA, Naseem S (2006) Oral submucous fibrosis: a distressing disease with malignant potential. Indian J Community Med 31, 270-271.
56. Dyavanagoudai SN. Oral submucous fibrosis:Review on etiopathogenesis. J cancer sci Ther 2009;1:072-077.
57. Dietrich Hoffmann, Klaus D. Brunnemann, Bogdan Prokopczyk and MirjanaV. Djordjevic. Tobacco-specific N-nitrosamines and areca-derived N- nitrosamines: chemistry, biochemistry, carcinogrnicity and relevance to humans. J Toxic01 Environ Health 1994;41:1-52.
58. Shaik PS, Pachava S. the Role of vitamins and trace elements on oral health: A systemic review. Int J Med Rev 2017;4(1):22-31.

59. El-Labban NC, Canniff JP. Ultrastructural finding of Muscles degeneration in oral submucous fibrosis. J Oral Pathol;14:709-717.

60. Gupta SC, Signh M, Khanna S, Jain S. Oral Submucous fibrosis with possible effect on eustachian tube function: A tympanometric study. Indian J Otolaryngol Head Neck Surg 2004;56:183-5.

61. Shah M, Khatarkar A, Shah P, Alam N, Modh D. Tympanometric study of eustachian tube function in oral submucous fibrosis. Indian J Otol 2011;17:80- 2.

62. Siddiqui SN, Saawarn N, Nair PP, Singh P, Gharote HP, Hegde K. Eustachian tube dysfunction in OSMF- often present seldom discovered. J Clin Exp Dent. 2014 Oct1;6(4):e369-73.

63. Devi P, Sighn I, Setru R, Tyagi K, Singh D, Thiyam B. Evaluation of hearing deficit in patuents with oral submucous fibrosis. J Oral Sci. 2015; 57(2):109- 13.

64. Badra, D.S., Fathima, D., & Mahesh, D. Evaluation of Hearing Efficiency in Patients with Oral Sub mucous Fibrosis. Pharm. Sci. & Res. 2015.7(10):890- 892.

65. Sowbhagya. Audiometric and Tympanometric Assessment in Patients with Oral Submucous Fibrosis. British Journal of Medicine & Medical Research, 2016; 13(6): 1-7.

66. Chandran A, Aswath N. Assesment of function of Eustachian tube in oral submucous fibrosis – A Tympanometric study. Jour of clin and diag Res.2016: 10 : 13-15.

67. Kumar A. Effect of oral submucous fibrosis on Auditory tube function: A case control study. Int J Sci Stud 2018:6; 8-10

68. Gupta RP, Rai K, Hemani D, Gupta AK. A study of trace elements (copper and zinc) in oral submucous fibrosis. Indian J Otolaryngol.1987: 39, 104- 106.

69. Varghese, Sugathan CK, Balsubramanium G, Vijaykumar T. Serum copper and zinc levels in premalignant or malignant lesions of the oral cavity. Oncology 1987: 44(4): 224- 227.

70. Kumar A, Sharma SC, Sharma D, Chanra KC, Amit N et al. beneficial effect of oral zinc in the treatment of oral submucous fibrosis. Indian J. Pharmacol 1991: 23; 236- 241.

71. Cunningaiper DA. Studies on hematolofical profile and trace elements in oral submucous fibrosis. J clin. Biochem. Nutr 1995; 19:9 – 17.

72. Hebert JR, Gupta PC, Bhonsle RB, Mehta H, Zheng W, Sanderson M, Teas J.Dietary exposures and oral precancerous lesions in Srikakulam District, Andhra Pradesh, India. Public Health Nutr. 2002 Apr;5(2):303-12.
73. Master Luquman, Vishnudas Dinesh, Prabhu, Vidya M. The role of serum copper and Iron in oral submucous fibrosis. JIAOMR 2004:16;30- 32
74. Khanna SS, Karjodkar FR. Circulating immune complexes and trace elements (Copper, Iron and Selenium) as markers in oral precancer and cancer : a randomised, controlled clinical trial. Head Face Med. 2006 Oct 16;2:33.
75. Nayak A, Kanthchatra L, Shenai PK. Analysis of copper and zinc levels in the mucosal tissue and serum of oral submucous fibrosis patients. World JDent. 2010;1:75-78
76. Shettar SS, Mubeen. Estimation of Serum Copper and Zinc Levels in Patients with Oral Submucous Fibrosis. J Indian acad oral med Radiol. 2010;22(4):193-196
77. Balpande A, Sathwane RS. Estimation of copper, zinc and copper / zinc ratio in oral leukoplakia, oral submucous fibrosis and squamous cell carcinoma. JIAOMR. 2010; 22(2); 73-76.
78. Ray JG, Ghosh R, Malick D, Gandhi NP. Correlation of Trace elemental profiles in blood samples of Indian patients with leukoplakia. Biol Trace Elem Res. 2011;011:90-91.
79. Ganapathy KS, Gurudath S, Balikai B, Ballal S, Sujatha D. Role of Iron deficiency in oral submucous fibrosis: an initiation and accelerating factor. JIAOMR 2011;23:25-28.
80. Tadakmadla J, Kumar S, Mamatha GP. Evaluation of serum copper and Iron levels amoung oral submucous fibrosis patients. Med Oral Patol Oral Cir Bucal. 2011 Nov 1;16 (7):870-3.
81. Ayinampudi BK, Narsmhan M. Salivary copper and zinc levels in oral premalignant and malignant lesions.J Oral MaxillofacPathol 2012;16:178-82.
82. Shetty SR, Babu S , Kumari S , Shetty P , et al Evaluation of micronutrient status in serum and saliva of oral submucous fibrosis patients: a clinicopathlogical study . Indian J Med Paediatr Oncol 2012;33:224-6.
83. Hegde K, Nair P, Gharote HP, Agarwal K, 1 Bhat GP, Rajaram DK. Role of Hemoglobin and Serum Iron in Oral Submucous Fibrosis: A Clinical Study. ScientificWorldJournal. 2012

84. Kamath VV, Satelur K, Komali Y. Biochemical markers in oral submucous fibrosis. A Review and update.Dent Res J 2013;10:576-84.

85. Shetty SR, Babu S, Kumari S, Shetty P , Hegde S, Karikal, A. Role of Serum Trace Elements in Oral Precancer and Oral Cancer - A biochemical study. J Cancer Res. Treat. 2013:1(1);1-3.

86. Kapoor S, Kaur M, Dangi CBS et al. Quantitative analysis of trace elements and heamoglobin as biological marker in patients with oral submucous fibrosis in central India. The Journal of Public Health. Photon 2013:115;147-158.

87. Kode MA, Karjodkar FR. Estimation of the Serum and the Salivary Trace Elements in OSMF Patients. J Clin Diagn Res. 2013 Jun;7(6):1215-8.

88. Neethi H, Patil S, Rao RS. Estimation of serum copper and zinc levels in oral submucous fibrosis: An atomic absorption soectroscopic study. J ClinDiagn Res. 2013: Vol-7(6): 1215-1218.

89. Sunali Khanna, A.C. Udas, G. Kiran Kumar, S Suvarna, FR Khajodkar. Trace elements (Copper, Zinc, Selenium and Molybdenum) as markers in oral submucous fibrosis and Oral squamous cell carcinoma. J Trace Elem MediBio 2013;27:307–311

90. Hosthor SS, Mahesh P, Priya SA, Sharada P, Jyotsna M, Chitra S. Quantitative analysis of serum levels of trace elements in patients with oral submucous fibrosis and oral squamous cell carcinoma: A randomized cross- sectional study. J Oral Maxillofac Pathol. 2014 Jan;18(1):46-51

91. Guruprasad R, Nair PP, Singh M, Singh MP, Jain A. serum vitamin C and iron levels in oral submucous fibrosis. Indian J Dent 2014;5:81-5.

92. Mohammad F, Manohar V, Jose M, Fairozekhan A, Mohamed S, Shamaz BH et al. Estimation of copper in saliva and areca nut products and its correlation with histological grades of orallsubmucos fibrosis. J Oral Pathol Med (2015) 44: 208–213.

93. Shetty SR, Babu S, Kumari S, Shetty P, Hegde S, Karikal A. status of trace elemts in saliva of oral precancer and oral cancer patients. J Can Res 2015;11:146-9.

94. Hammed F, Ali I, Khan, Aqeel Aslam M, Haeez N, Haider SM et al.Estimation of serum iron in oral submucous fibrosis patients and its comparison with healthy controls.PakistanJOtolaryngol 2015; 43-46.

95. Saurabh S, Sunil MK, Kumar R, Mishra A,Birring OJ, Khan L. Estimation of serum iron & protein levels in oral submucous fibrosis: A clinical research. J Med RadiolPathol Surg 2015;1:3-6.

96. Yadav A, Kumar L, Misra N, Deepak U, ShivKumar GC. Estimation of serum zinc, copper and iron in the patients of oral submucous fibrosis. Natl J Maxillofac Surg 2015;6:190-3.

97. Srilekha M. Copper and Zinc level in oral submucous fibrosis (OSMF) patients. J. Pharm. Sci. & Res. 2015:7(8); 573-574.

98. Okade AR, Hallikeri KS, Trivedi DJ. Salivary Estimation of copper iron zinc and manganese in oral submucous fibrosis patient. Clin cancer investing J 2015;4:302-6.

99. Tiwari R, David CM, Mahesh DR, Sambargi U, Rashmi KJ, Benakanal P. Assessment of serum copper, iron and immune complexes in potentially malignant disorders and oral cancer. Braz Oral Res. 2016 Oct 10;30(1):e101.

100. Bhardwaj D, Dinkar AD, Satoskar SK, Desai SR. Serum Iron and Haemoglobin estimation in oral submucous fibrosis and iron deficiency anemia: A Diagnostic approach. J Clin Diagn Res. 2016;10(12):54-58.

101. Kallali BN, Gujjar PK, Rawson K, Bhalerao S, Pereira T, Zingade J. Analysis of iron levels in the mucosal tissue and serum of oral submucous fibrosis patients.J Indian Acad Oral Med Radiol 2016;28:119-23.

102. Kumar H, Kumar P, Jain S, Suryawanshi H. Analysis of serum Copper and Iron Levels in Oral submucous fibrosis patients: a Case-Control Study. Indian J dent sci 2016;8:145-9.

103. More C.B, Patel H. Trace elements in potentially oral malignant disorders and oral malignant lesion- A biochemical study. Int J Ora Max Dis; 1(2); 2016:1-7.

104. Thakur M, Guttikonda VR. Estimation of haemoglobin, serum iron, total iron binding capacity and serum ferritin levels in oral submucous fibrosis: A clinicopathalogical Study. J Oral Maxillofac Pathol 2017;21:30-5.

105. Latoo S, Nazil H. Estimation of levels of copper and iron in different stages of OSMF Patients. Ann of Int. Med and Dent Resea. 2017: 3(5).

106. Jayi YV, Chaudhary AR, Dudhia BB, Bhatia PV, Soni NC, Patel PS. Evaluation of role of trace elements in oral submucous fibrosis patients : A study on Gujarati Population. J Oral Maxillofac Pathol 2017;21:455.

107. Bhalerao SM, Lohe VK, Bhowate RR. Estimation of Iron and Vitamin C levels in serum and saliva: A clinic and biochemical study in oral submucous fibrosis patients. Ann. Int. Med. Den. Res. 2018; 4(3):43-53.

108. K Ranganathan. Mishra Gauri. An overview of classification schemes for oral submucous fibrosis. J Oral Maxillofac Pathol.2006;10(2):55-58.

109. G.P Butrimovitz and W.C Purdy G. P. The determination of zinc in Blood Plasma By Atomic Absorption spectrophotometry. Anal. Chim. Acta 94, 63 (1977).

110. J.B Dawson, D.J Ellis, H. Newton-John. Direct Estimation of copper in serum and Urine by Atomic absorption spectroscopy. Clin. Chim. Acta 21,33 (1968).

111. A.D Olson, W.B Hamlin. A new method for serum iron and total iron binding capacity by atomic absorption spectrophotometry. Clin. Chem. 15, 438 (1969).

112. Haider SM, Merchant AT, Fikree FF, Rahbar MH. Clinical and Functional staging of oral submucous fibrosis. Br J Oral Maxillofac Surg. 2000;38:12-5.

113. Gupta SC. Clay induced oral submucous fibrosis. Gupta SC. Clay induced oral submucous fibrosis. Indian J orolaryngol 1987:39 28.

114. Binnie WH, Cowson RA. A new ultrastructural finding in oral submucous fibrosis. Br J dermatol 1972:86;286

115. Oliver AJ, Radden BG. Oral submucous fibrosis. Case report and review of literature. Aust Dent J. 1992;37:31-4.

116. Rajendra R. Oral submucous fibrosis. J Oral Maxillofac Pathol. 2003;7:1-4.

117. Fong LY, Riley M, Farber JL. Zinc deficiency promotes cancer of the upper aerodigestive tract (UDAT) by activation of NF-kB and COX-2. Proc Amer Assoc Cancer Res 2006;66(8);746.

118. Katharia SK, Singh SP, Kulshreshtha VK. The effects of Placenta extract in management of oral submucous fibrosis. Indian J pharmacol 1992;24;181-83.

Kolibri 360 GmbH
Ferdinand-Jühlke-Straße 7
99095 Erfurt, Deutschland
produktsicherheit@kolibri360.de

Druck:
CPI Druckdienstleistungen GmbH
im Auftrag der
Kolibri 360 GmbH
Ferdinand-Jühlke-Str. 7
99095 Erfurt